365 Daily Meditations

for On and Off the Mat

A Year in Hot Yoga

SCOTT GINSBERG

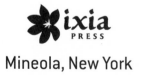

ixia
PRESS

Mineola, New York

This book is a love letter and thank-you note to the amazing students, teachers, owners, staff, and work-study volunteers at *Yoga Tribe Brooklyn.* You are my family, my center of belonging, my group therapy, and my favorite place to be. Namaste.

Bibliographical Note

365 Daily Meditations for On and Off the Mat: A Year in Hot Yoga
is a new work, first published by Ixia Press in 2017.

International Standard Book Number

ISBN-13: 978-0-486-81693-7
ISBN-10: 0-486-81693-1

IXIA PRESS
An imprint of Dover Publications, Inc.

Manufactured in the United States by LSC Communications
81693101   2017
www.doverpublications.com/ixiapress

January 1

Begin a ritual that reflects your needs.

The first day of the year is always one of my favorite times to go to yoga class. People slouch into the studio tired and hungover, still absolutely committed to starting their year off on the right foot. The room is always crowded, full of old friends and eager new faces, all wanting a fresh wave of momentum as the year kicks off.

Meanwhile, reporters tell us that the majority of adults who make annual fitness resolutions give up within a few months. Their pessimism sends the message that we should give up and realize that we're powerless to alter our situation. But assuming failure only guarantees that we'll never get started. The trick is to find a routine and goal that actually works for you. Personally, hot yoga was different for me. Unlike other fitness regimens or healthy practices, it was astounding how easy it was to stick with it. Showing up and sweating out the postures quickly became a "must," not a "should." It became a ritual that reflected and shaped my deeply held values. As a result, yoga became something that wasn't worth missing, instead of something that flamed out in a flash of the pan.

If you want to start the year off strong, ignore the articles and news reports forecasting the doom and gloom of resolution abandonment. That's all just noise. We don't need to believe naysayers or assume that we're doomed to be part of the percentage who flunks out of their resolutions. Keep your head down, figure out what your standards are, create rituals around them, and start your journey. You've got this.

 How will you defy the odds this year?

January 2

You can fall, as long as you get up again.

The first time I took hot yoga, I slipped on my mat and nearly fell on my butt. Instead of embarrassing me in front of the class, my instructor gently remarked: "Thank you for listening to your body."

I felt more encouraged immediately. She wasn't critical; she was appraising. She wasn't harsh; she was constructive. She wasn't frustrated; she was supportive. And she wasn't judgmental; she was thankful. It was an act of spirit in a moment of struggle.

 How do you respond to yourself when you fall down?

January 3

Check your baggage.

A common question that new yoga students ask is what they should bring to their first class. Easy answer: A towel, mat, water, and some lightweight clothing. Then again, all of those items can be bought or borrowed at the yoga studio, if need be. The real question first-time students should be asking is, what should I *not* bring to class?

That's probably more helpful. Enjoying class will be much easier if you experience it with a blank slate, free of your weighty preconceptions. In fact, there should be a sign at the entrance to every yoga studio for the attention of all new students: "To get the most out of today's class, please leave the following items outside the door: your ego, your expectations, your perfectionism, any judgments about yourself, all competitive urges about others, and whatever other mental rubbish you'd like to dispose of. Namaste."

 What are you bringing into the room that doesn't belong?

January 4

A flexible body changes everything.

Often we seek out yoga to expand our range of motion after an injury, for postpartum recovery, or just to create a better baseline for our fitness. It might be that you want to manage or prevent arthritis, and that the rest of the practice is an afterthought. But flexibility is more than physical. There is mental, spiritual, and life flexibility as well.

Sure, I can reach my toes and touch my head to my knees. But the capacity to respond flexibly to what the world hurls at me? The ability to entertain ideas completely contrary to my own? The patience to sit quietly next to someone who drives me crazy?

We all know the saying that God laughs when we make plans. Adjusting to that disruption requires a completely different kind of flexibility, one that yoga can help you develop. Your body affects every other life experience you have. Stretch your muscles and you stretch your life.

 How can you increase your flexibility?

January 5

The only equipment you need is yourself.

Unlike many physical activities, yoga requires no equipment beyond the readiness to practice it. You don't need the sexy outfit or the perfect mat or the deluxe thermos to begin. Those are just containers into which you pour procrastination or inflate your ego. Convenient excuses you make for not showing up to do the real work.

At our studio, we have a community lost-and-found bin. It's a treasure trove of mats, towels, shorts, shirts, water bottles, and other accessories people have accidentally left behind. What's nice is that if you show up to class and realize that you've forgotten something, you're welcome to dig through the bin and borrow whatever you need.

I remember working the front desk one afternoon when a new student showed up completely unprepared for his very first class. No workout clothes, no water bottle, no nothing. He felt terrible, to the point that he considered leaving the studio and coming back another time. I told him: don't let this be the reason you miss class today. You're already here. Just go grab some extra clothes from the lost-and-found and do the best you can. The other students will be too focused on their own practice to even notice you anyway. The guy smiled, said thanks, and agreed to stick around. Five minutes later, he was on the mat, sweating with the rest of us, practicing his first-ever hot yoga class. And even though he was wearing someone else's clothes, he did the best he could. Not because he had the right equipment, but because he had the readiness to practice. That's how yoga works. Bring the right attitude to it, and the rest will follow.

 What excuses can you overcome today?

January 6

Don't make a global judgment from a single effort.

If you think your first hot yoga class was hard, don't let it keep you from your second one. It will be light-years easier. Because this time, you know what to expect. You also know how to prepare.

That's why teachers tell new students to return within twenty-four hours. The sooner you come back for your second class, the better. It helps your body acclimate to the heat faster, bypass much of the muscle soreness, and ultimately help you decide if the practice is right for you.

Which it might not be. With hot yoga, people seem to either love it or hate it. And that's fine. But like a lot of new habits, it won't stick right away. In fact, you might not even be ready for it the first few tries. Every day your body is different. It takes at least two, maybe three, classes before you can make an informed decision. Had I created an impression about hot yoga from my pathetic first class performance, I never would have returned. Good thing I came back and gave it another chance.

 Are you allowing yourself to give up before it gets good?

January 7

Dive in without reservations.

So often we wait endlessly to be "ready." One of our teachers has an inspiring mantra for beginning students: Move the muscles whether you feel ready or not.

This directive is helpful when you're struggling in postures because it challenges you to trust your own body. For example, balancing poses like tree and triangle require significant shifts of body weight onto your feet and toes. It can be scary when everyone around you is executing the postures beautifully. I've certainly felt inadequate when compared to some of the twenty-year veterans at my studio.

The best part about practicing yoga is just that—it's practice. You can experiment with moving your muscles, despite your lack of vast expertise. Inch by inch, day by day, until you're suddenly touching your nose to your knee and feeling like a superstar. You won't start out there, but you do have to start somewhere in order to advance to a higher level.

 When was the last time you took the leap of trusting that you were ready to handle something new and scary?

January 8

Allow life to show you the new way to move forward.

When we first start practicing yoga, there's a lot of newness. New feelings, new thoughts, new positions, new lessons, even new parts of the body that we didn't know we had. This uncertainty, uncomfortable as it may be, shows up to teach us a more meaningful lesson. My yoga instructor said it best one morning: *Instead of questioning what this experience is, just receive it.*

What a difficult thing for us to do. We're addicted to naming, organizing, labeling, and understanding every experience we have. Anything less offends our sense of order and control. God forbid we simply allow something to happen to us. God forbid we accept whatever feelings arise. God forbid that we don't know why or what something is.

It's scary to cede control and knowledge over a situation, which is why we resist it. But yoga insists that we let go. Inside and outside of class, we learn to release our grip on the known and open our hands to receive the new.

 Are you missing out on the benefits of yoga by wanting to already have mastery?

January 9

Better to miss a posture than to make yourself sick.

The first few classes of hot yoga can be overwhelming. With the heat and physical exertion, you might even feel dizzy or a bit nauseous. It's normal. Happens every day around the world, to newbies and veterans alike. As most instructors will tell you, sitting out is not only accepted, but also encouraged. Just do the best you can. If you feel overwhelmed, take a break. Rejoin the group when you're ready.

It sounds nice in the abstract, but there's an inner dilemma. After all, you paid for the class, so there's financial guilt; a certified instructor is teaching you, so there are power dynamics; you have a room full of experienced students, so there's social pressure; and you have your own ego, so there are feelings involving shame and pride and failure.

Do yourself a favor and put aside those influences and listen to yourself.

 What nonexistent rules are you afraid to break?

January 10

Don't rush yourself.

During our first few yoga classes, we're likely to look at the clock repeatedly, wondering to ourselves, *when is this torture going to end?*

What we learn after practicing for a while is that we can't move through the postures faster than the hands of the clock will allow. That's part of the yoga. Maturing our sense of time. Learning how to surrender to the moment and forget about the clock. My teacher has this great saying: *Wonder when the posture is over by breathing.*

In other words, channel your anxiety into a more productive and present activity. Slip away from the domain of the clock by focusing on your inhales and exhales, and you'll float away to that lovely, timeless world inside your body. Just remember, regardless of what the clock says, there's always plenty of time to listen to your inner voice.

 Was the clock ticking loudly, or was that just my heart expanding?

January 11

Take a pose of empowerment.

Showing up and doing postures each day gives me an arena to practice choosing how to relate to my body, my mind, my soul, my ambition, my community, and my space. And that's just during the warm-up.

Throughout class, a vast new world of other choices begins to unfold. Like the choice to let the sweat drip and not wipe it away every five seconds. Because each time I witness myself choosing, there's a part of me that says, Wow, I wonder what else I am able to make choices about.

Choice is perhaps the greatest power of all. Choosing to execute movements your own way, whether stretching your hands to the ceiling or wringing out your spine like a wet rag—these actions build a foundation that ripples out into the rest of our lives.

 Now that you've made this choice, what else might you be able to make choices about?

January 12

Save your energy for your practice.

During yoga class, my obsessive-compulsive tendencies often come crashing to the surface. Like when my towel and mat aren't perfectly ironed out and parallel with the mirror. That bothers me. It offends my sense of order. To the point that it becomes one of those annoying itches that I can't help but scratch.

Whoops, let me just straighten this little wrinkle here—should only take a second.

I interrupt the posture and engage in a little housekeeping project on my mat until everything is right with the world again. My instructor actually called me out on it the other day. He stared at me and said:

Scott, your mat and towel-straightening skills are not going to improve.

Busted. I was wasting my energy on the wrong activity. One that paid no dividends, distracted the other students in the class, and triggered my obsessive-compulsive behaviors. That's not why you pay twenty dollars a class. The goal is to deepen your practice, not get better at folding laundry.

 How often does your mind carry you off to a fantasyland of compulsion and control?

January 13

A wave of peacefulness.

Can doing yoga make you a more peaceful person? Maybe. Throw a rock and you can find any number of studies, some from rigorous randomized, controlled trials, showing that yoga may help reduce stress and anxiety and also enhance your mood and overall sense of well-being. But if your expectation is that yoga will somehow bring you into a lifelong state of complete mental serenity free from any stress or anxiety, it might be time to wake up. Life will still hold surprises and set you off-kilter.

The difference is having tools to cope. Personally, practicing yoga did teach me how to find and develop my own internal supply of peace within the practice. When life starts ratcheting up its level of tension and stress, it's simply a matter of transporting yourself back to that internal supply of peace. Because the body never forgets. We can draw from the feeling of completion and serenity that arrives after finishing a pose.

We can't stay within that calm forever, but we can grow the ability to find our way back to a condition of peace whenever we have lost it. We advance in our lessened attachment to each mental state, which makes it easier for us to let go of passing irritations.

 How has doing yoga changed your relationship with peace?

January 14

Abandon expectations.

Lately I've been learning new ways to treat myself with compassion and patience. How to meet more and more of my life experiences with kindness and understanding. It's been an enlightening and rewarding journey. One practice I find to be particularly helpful is abandoning expectations about how I'm supposed to feel. Especially when it comes to my goals and dreams. Because when I first write them down, I tend to create this fantasy in my head about how things are going to be better when they come to pass. About how I'm going to know a different kind of happiness that I've never known before.

But it doesn't always happen like that. Even though we wait for that one huge life moment with fireworks and banners and trombones, most goals and dreams unfold slowly and quietly. And we get outraged when we can't impose our own time frame on the process. Doing our yoga postures works the same way. It's the danger of harboring expectations about how things should go that disrupts them. White-knuckling and trying to control the outcome only leads to disappointment.

If we want to free ourselves from the clutches of unnecessary distress, we have to be compassionate and accepting of the results we get. In the *Bhagavad Gita,* Krishna said that we have a right to our labor, but not to the fruits of our labor. That's the approach we have to take with our daily life, on or off the mat. Focus on the intention of the execution, and let the rest go.

 What expectations are you prepared to abandon?

January 15

Acclimate to even the most unpleasant conditions.

One element that attracted me to hot yoga was the satisfaction of expelling massive amounts of sweat from my body. In the ninety minutes of my very first class, I could literally feel my pores cleansing and stress releasing. There was so much sweat, the blue dye ran right out of my shorts and stained my towel. It was glorious. Few other forms of exercise offer such a unique experience. Of course, many people avoid hot yoga for this very reason. The sloppiness of the practice triggers their inner germophobe, and the lack of personal space offends their sense of order.

It makes sense. None of us enjoys getting sweat flung into our eye from a half-naked stranger. But if you ask people who are committed to the practice, although they might not love the sweat, they do accept it. Maybe they even miss it when it's been a few days or a few weeks since their last practice.

It sounds a bit gross, but if hot yoga teaches us anything, it's the ability of the human mind and body to acclimate to even the most unpleasant conditions. If the first Noble Truth of Buddhism is that "Life is suffering," perhaps getting used to minor discomforts will pay dividends in increasing our resilience against larger ones.

 What is something that you used to think was impossible and has now become strangely enjoyable?

January 16

Accept yourself as you are.

During my first month of yoga many years ago, I recall the teacher telling our class the following: Look at yourself in the mirror without judgment. As a reflection and nothing else. There's nothing to change or fix or heal or improve. Just notice it.

I was sold. For me, being something of a perfectionist, the message was radical. Never before had I been given permission or space to be open to all that I am. Too often, the message is about contorting ourselves to be different, or "better." With yoga, we achieve freedom to merely be.

 Do you see yourself as you are or as you want yourself to be?

January 17

Drop the demands.

When I get upset with my yoga instructors, it's usually because they fail to fulfill an assignment that I have mentally given them. Can't they read my mind? Satisfy my implicit demands? Live up to my unrealistic expectations? To my frustration, they can't. That's not how the teacher/student relationship, or any relationship for that matter, works. Just because I prefer to have the yoga room as hot and humid and swampy as possible doesn't mean the instructor will read my mind and promptly crank up the thermostat and close the windows.

Sometimes, that's my practice for the day: In all of my relationships, accepting that the world does not revolve around me. Remembering that people aren't here to facilitate my precious little preferences.

 Which of your expectations have become demands?

January 18

Absorb some of the weight-bearing responsibility.

Here's something my yoga teacher recently asked the class during a difficult balancing pose: If the floor disappeared right now, which muscles would you be engaging?

It's a tough question because it confronts us with one of our unconscious yoga habits, gripping the floor with our fingers or toes to maintain balance. Although it's tempting to do so, it's just a crutch. The floor shouldn't be the thing we depend on, our body should be.

Instead of turning our limbs into fleshy vise-like grips, it's smarter to engage the core and flex the surrounding muscle groups. This creates a durable foundation that absorbs some of the weight-bearing responsibility from our fingers and toes. When you're strong in your center, you don't need to hang on so desperately at the edges.

 What unconscious yoga habits are you trying to break?

January 19

Build your inner six-pack.

Yoga helps us build muscles we didn't know we had, like the ones in our feet, hips, lower back, neck, and fingers. Yoga also helps build muscles we didn't know were muscles, like patience, stillness, forgiveness, courage, respect, and acceptance.

Unfortunately, none of these muscles makes us look better in our swimsuits. They don't give us the beach body we so badly crave. And they won't increase our chances of getting picked as a contestant on that new modeling reality show. But building these muscles *will* make us love ourselves and others more. No spray tan needed.

 What unexpected benefits has yoga given you?

January 20

Stop trying to control appearances.

If students are trying to look good in front of each other, yoga won't work. If people are denying vulnerability to maintain face, yoga won't work. And if people are addicted to curating a specific self-image, yoga won't work.

Only when we finally break free of the constant pressure to perform can we build deep connection and true intimacy. Only when we accept that it's okay not to be okay can we grow together. And you can't learn that lesson if you're too busy putting on a show for people.

We fight this battle in our minds in yoga class every day. It's hard to look into the mirror and accept our own flaws, *without* comparing our bodies to other students. The secret is to offer a gift to others by being courageously vulnerable and showing the more tender aspects of who we are. Even if our yoga pants don't fit as perfectly as those on the person practicing next to us. Drop the façade and try being real at last.

 Once you liberate yourself from keeping up with appearances, what might be possible for you?

January 21

All battles are internal.

Bikram Yoga founder Bikram Chaudhury's philosophy on yoga is that it's just you, and nothing but you. Standing in one spot frozen like a statue with no place to go for help, except inward. It's challenging work. Most people aren't used to, or ready for, that level of confrontation with the self. The inclination is to look for excuses or scapegoats. That's just blame-shifting. All battles, whether won or lost, are internal. It's always you versus you.

In *Rocky IV,* Rocky Balboa asks this very question about a fight: *Do you think maybe it ain't against him? Do you think maybe it's you against you?* Apollo Creed responds dismissively, but the champ was right. Whatever battle we're fighting, on the mat, in the ring, or out in the world, it's always the human heart in conflict with itself.

 How have you been avoiding confronting yourself?

January 22

Make your habit historic.

Our personhood is carved out by the flow of our habits. If we want to engrave our desired behaviors so deeply that they become natural and instinctual, we have to make space to integrate them into our lives.

I'm reminded of a useful mantra that my yoga instructor recites at the end of each class. Give your body time to memorize the new habits you started, she says. Luxuriate for a few minutes. Soak it all in. That way, next time you come in to practice, muscle memory will engage, and you'll perform the postures with less conscious awareness.

That's how habit grows. It needs space. David Brooks's book *The Road to Character* takes it one step further. His research into history's great achievers suggests that we make the beginning of a new habit a major event in our lives. This way we launch with as strong and decisive an initiative as possible. Whatever new habit you intend to start, make it momentous. Do something tangible, memorable, and public. Throw a party, write a press release, or email twenty friends to commemorate your start on this journey. By raising the significance attached to the habit, you guard yourself against anything that might weaken it in the future.

 How will you announce your intentions to the universe?

January 23

Allow time for self-care.

Recently the Veterans Administration has been experimenting with using yoga for the treatment of veterans. It turns out that there is a growing openness to complementary and integrative medicine in the medical field. Not only is yoga used for the retired military personnel themselves, it's also been used for the healthcare providers who care for the patients. Pamela Pence, a yoga teacher involved in one of the trials, said the following:

> As caregivers, it's an honor to be on the journey with these veterans. But working in a military hospital environment can be overwhelming when you are witness to the challenges faced by veterans in their daily lives. It is essential to maintain a steady personal yoga practice to avoid taking on the suffering of others and to allow you to serve sustainably.

It's a modern version of the ancient saying: *Quis custodiet ipsos custodes?* Meaning: who guards the guards? Who cares for the caregivers? If you work in a helping profession, make sure you're taking the time to care for your own needs. Work on your postures so you can help other people with theirs.

 What would a high level of self-care be for you?

January 24

Allow yoga to set its own limits.

Our edge is the best place to learn about ourselves. The challenge is approaching that place with safety, intention, and grace. During a recent posture clinic, a visiting instructor offered a great piece of advice about this process:

> *If you're trying to push yourself past where you are honestly able to go, you will no longer be practicing yoga, but practicing greed. Let the yoga surprise you. Allow it to set its own limits, rather than trying to impose limits on your own based on what you think you should do.*

It's an exercise in active listening. Not the kind of "listening" in which we make eye contact and nod and parrot words back to the speaker. But the kind where we take action on our body's intuitive leads, following sensations all the way to our limit without the compulsion to push ourselves past it.

 What have you learned about yourself at the edge?

January 25

Permission to opt out.

What if I can't do all of the poses? Good question. The simple answer is: *don't*. It's a freeing word. Despite our fears, there are no yoga police coming to kick down the door and confiscate your mat.

It's perfectly appropriate for even longtime practitioners to take a break during class. Sit out as long as you'd like. The stillness allows you to regain breath and composure, and to try again once you've recovered. In fact, the only crime students can commit is trying to soldier on with the posture, in pain and out of fear. That's where injuries, dehydration, and scathing online reviews come from.

If yoga gets a bit overwhelming, don't be too scared to give up the task for a moment and allow yourself the space you need. Your mat isn't going anywhere. It'll be there when you're ready to return.

 How would your practice be different if you accepted that you don't have to do everything right, or at all?

January 26

Breathe through the pain.

During some of the longer postures in yoga, I frequently find myself struggling. It's amazing how long sixty seconds feels when you're doing a full backbend in hundred-degree heat. Fortunately, there is a secret to holding those lengthy poses. Let your body do the one thing it naturally does best: Breathe.

There's no better way to center yourself. Plus, breathing helps you reignite momentum from a relaxed, nondestructive space. Sadly, most people lose touch with their breathing. Then they clumsily plunge forward from a place of contraction and fear. If you feel yourself flagging, breathe into the moment to find your center. It's something you can apply on the yoga mat or off.

 How's your breathing?

January 27

Appreciate your freedom to breathe.

We all define freedom in our own way. As we should. That's the whole point of being free in the first place. Singer-songwriter Kris Kristofferson sang that "freedom's just another name for nothing left to lose." My definition is simpler. To me, freedom is the ability to breathe. It's that blissful state of psychological sovereignty in which the pressures of life aren't constricting your life force into a distracted haze, and you can finally just be here now and touch real joy. You can breathe and revel in the gentle restfulness and slow lightness of being.

I only know this because I've experienced the opposite. When I was twenty-six, I suffered a collapsed lung. I got up one morning, couldn't breathe, went to the emergency room, woke up a few hours later with a tube in my chest, and then spent a week in the hospital connected to a respirator that did my breathing for me. It was the polar opposite of freedom.

My suffering wasn't special. People's lungs collapse every day, and in most cases, treatment is fairly simple: Oxygen and rest. However, that experience fundamentally changed me forever. It was the inciting incident that led me to yoga. For the past ten years, that practice has given me a deeper understanding and appreciation of one of the most basic freedoms we have as human beings. *Breathing. Inhaling. Exhaling.* Sometimes it takes losing something to appreciate having it in the first place.

 How do you define freedom?

January 28

Don't fight reality during the postures.

Directly above my yoga studio is a fitness boot camp. People flip tractor tires and drag chains across the floor, while the instructor shouts slogans at them until they eventually crumple to the floor in a puddle of sweat and tears. It's a challenge to meditate and stay focused in yoga postures. If you're not used to it, the thuds and vibrations can be highly distracting to your postures.

One night there was a new student practicing on the mat to my left whose patience was wearing thin. Each time somebody from the boot camp crashed down on the floor above us, he would look up at the ceiling with a withering scowl. Ten minutes into class, he couldn't take it anymore. He ripped his mat and towel off the floor, stormed out of class in a fury of frustration, and immediately exited the studio. So much for using yoga as a vehicle for transformation and peace.

It was a powerful lesson for the rest of the students in the room, a reminder that frustration comes from our refusal to accept life's moments as they come to us. Our job, whether we're practicing yoga or not, is to love and even laugh at those distractions, instead of waging a campaign against them. Buddhist teacher and author Pema Chödrön's advice on staying sane during difficult times makes the point that pain comes from holding so tightly to having it our own way. Don't march out of the room in a huff every time the vibrations of the world throw your posture off balance.

 Have you learned how to relate sanely during difficult times?

January 29

Make zero demands.

I once overheard a first-time yoga student make a list of demands for the instructor before class started. It was mind-blowing. She explained that she didn't like the room too hot, insisted on placing her mat by the back door, didn't want any individual attention or corrections from the teacher, and had to duck out fifteen minutes early. Well then. That's certainly *one* type of posture.

It was a helpful reminder for my own practice. Anytime we walk into a room with our own personal hospitality rider, we're only setting ourselves up for disappointment. In my perfect world, every yoga studio would be legally obligated to post the following disclaimer: *What should you expect when you come to our studio? Nothing.*

You'll have the best class of your life.

 Are you learning to make fewer unrealistic demands on yourself and others?

January 30

Beating yourself up during class? Don't.

When we first start practicing yoga, we want to excel. If we slip and fall during class or confront a challenging backbend, we assume that something must have gone horribly wrong. But it's simply life doing what it does. We need to accept the fact that, along with the billions of other people on the planet, we're imperfect individuals, just as likely as anyone else to be hit by the slings and arrows of outrageous, but perfectly normal, misfortune.

Buddhists and Hindus call this approach to life *maitri* or *mettā*, which centers on developing loving kindness in our unconditional friendship with ourselves. That means putting an end to some of our unhealthier habits. Such as heaping blame on ourselves when we stumble. Judging ourselves when we're wrong. Berating ourselves because we fall short of our high expectations. Whatever misfortune happens upon us, big or small, none of these reactions helps. If we're busy treating our mind like a battleground where we tear ourselves up, *maitri* has no space in which to enter.

As usual, yoga postures are only microcosms of the larger postures of normal life. We must treat ourselves with unconditional positive regard when things don't go as well as we feel they should, on the mat and off.

 What's your most common way to beat yourself up during class?

January 31

Move through your feelings.

My bouts of sadness come and go. But the good news is, they're never debilitating, and they're always seasonal and situational. I never get so low that it becomes impossible for me to see anything beyond my current state, and I always believe in my bones that there is a tomorrow that can turn it all around. As my therapist once said, anxiety will get you out of bed, depression will keep you in it.

In fact, I'm secretly grateful for my times of sadness. I often have the strongest, most enlightening yoga classes during those periods: they are the moments when the magic is trying to enter. Holocaust survivor Viktor Frankl observed that as soon as a painful fate cannot be changed, it must not only be accepted, but transmuted into something meaningful.

It's a two-part process. First, notice and name any feelings of sadness, honoring them with the attention they deserve; and second, start creating with whatever energy is inside of you. Even if it's blocked energy, it's still energy, which means we can use it.

 What do you do with your feelings?

February 1

Anyone can meditate on a mountain.

In the same way that we don't get credit for cleaning up our own mess, we don't get it for extending compassion to people we like. As we say in class, *anybody can meditate on a mountain.* Meaning, our effort only counts when it's hard.

Working as a volunteer at my yoga studio helped train my heart in this regard. Every day, you're assigned a random assortment of humanity. In any public-facing role, there are personalities and attitudes and behaviors that make you want to run away when you see them coming. In those times, compassion asks us to stay in the room. To build patience and space for everybody's dysfunctions. Someone who drives us crazy might simply be a good person trapped inside bad behavior, fighting a battle that we know nothing about.

This expression of compassion makes for more loving interactions, more welcoming communities, and more loyal relationships. Not just inside a beautiful yoga studio where everything is soothing and warm, but out in the world where it's often cold and cruel. Because that's where people need it the most.

 How much compassion do you have for people who have been sent to teach you about love?

February 2

Are you a hypocrite, or just human?

All yogis have their current favorite and least favorite posture. These may change quite frequently, based on your body, your attitude, your needs, and the seasons of life in which you practice. One day you're foaming at the mouth to execute a backbend, open up your thoracic cavity, and make your tender bits vulnerable to the world; the next month you're scared and tired and want nothing more than to cradle yourself in child's pose and never come out.

The key is to not beat yourself up for these fluctuations. To be alive in all your contradictions. Because contradiction doesn't mean you are a hypocrite, only that you're a growing, moving, imperfect human being taking new shape and form every time you step onto the mat. Historian Daniel Boorstin said it best: "Learning, I have found, is a way of becoming inconsistent with my past self."

 Are you accepting your humanity during class?

February 3

Question the commercialization of your practice.

Yoga has had a profound effect on my life. The practice has transformed my life in numerous ways, from physically to emotionally to spiritually. However, in my ten years as a student, I have never once considered investing any time, money, effort, or emotional energy in the process of acquiring the perfect yoga mat. It's neither here nor there as a feature that supports my yoga practice.

For some the yoga mat is more than just a tool; it's also a symbol and a sacred space and, in many cases, a reflection of the student's personality and practice. That's a beautiful notion. But let's not delude ourselves. Yoga has been around for five thousand years, whereas yoga mats have only been around for fifty. In that time, we've built a multibillion-dollar global yoga mat market predicated on people's desire to project the image of the ultimate yoga warrior.

It is, ironically, the exact opposite of yoga, a practice that's supposed to teach us presence and liberation. It's hard to rebel against the forces of attachment in our own hearts and surrender to joy in this moment if we're concerned with which brand of rubber we're standing on. The practice is not about the need to have the latest trend.

Remember, customer satisfaction is an oxymoron. That fancy yoga mat won't save you, won't make you happy, won't set you free, won't make you feel like you're enough, and won't be the one thing that changes everything. Let it go and enjoy the practice.

 What if you knew that nothing was missing right now?

February 4

Ignore your inner critic.

Every negative inner voice always starts as a negative outer voice. Somewhere down the line, you started to internalize the message of devaluation.

My yoga teacher once said that the most telling question he asked his students was: "Who was the first person in your life to tell you you weren't enough?" Moments like these never leave us, whether they come from parents, siblings, coaches, or friends.

The challenge, then, is to uncover the pivotal transition from outer voice to inner voice. To trace back to when we began internalizing a false story. For example, let's say that every time we eat ice cream after yoga class, there's a grating undercurrent of shame that keeps spoiling the joy of that experience.

Instead of judging ourselves, let's try to consider whose external voice we might be channeling. After all, our emotional reactions are based more on what *happened* to us than what's *happening* to us. In the process, we might discover that our negative emotional response to eating ice cream is quite reasonable based on our personal history. There's no need to shame ourselves every time we eat a chocolate-covered waffle cone with two scoops of peanut butter cookie dough and multicolored sprinkles.

If we're willing to plumb the depths of the self and uncover the origin of our most insidious critical voices, we're likely to discover that they're not even ours in the first place. That frees us to ignore them and focus on listening to our own voice.

 Are you assigning the proper relevance to your inner voice?

February 5

Take your practice as it comes.

Like any practice, yoga never stops evolving. Your mind, body, and soul are in one constant re-beginning. If you had a string of strong yoga classes where you felt unstoppable and focused during every posture, that's awesome. Well done. But don't be surprised if the following week, you suddenly feel rigid and weak and scatterbrained like a first-time student. It happens to the best of us, and it doesn't make you any more or less, any better or worse. Your practice is simply evolving. Remember that it's not about "perfecting" a pose but about continuing to seek.

 Which of your past successes are you afraid you can't duplicate?

February 6

Anxiety is a source of education.

Our main teacher is in the mirror. With it, the students' reflections become their own teachers. Yes, the instructor will help to keep the pace and make corrections, but ultimately, it's the process of confronting ourselves, warts and all, that activates real growth. Self-confrontation is a powerful tool to deepen your practice as a yoga student. It's a helpful lesson off the mat, too. Because that which is scariest to confront often has the most to teach us.

Philosopher Søren Kierkegaard referred to anxiety as the nameless and formless uneasiness that has dogged the footsteps of modern man. No wonder much of human behavior is motivated by a desire to escape anxiety. But let's not forget, anxiety is also a profound source of education for us. Just like the mirror in the yoga room, anxiety reflects our reality back to us.

Any time I feel anxiety hot on my trail, I try to reserve a small portion of my brain for gratitude. I give thanks for those feelings. Instead of treating the moment as if it were an obstacle to overcome, I use it as a vehicle to answer some questions about myself. To learn what might be lacking. To hear the story I've been telling myself about my own reality. More often than not, taking that small moment of awareness and curiosity leads me down a healthier path. One where I'm not averting my eyes from something in the mirror that I despise, but walking through the glass to see what lies on the other side.

 Are you willing to be your own best teacher?

February 7

Yoga is only practice.

The game we're training for is life. The good news is, the postures provide us with an intuitive structure that helps us more effectively meet the requirements of living. Our cardiovascular strength physically prepares us for the challenges we face later. Our flexibility mentally fortifies us against anything difficult that might happen the rest of the day. Our breathing skills allow us to solve problems as quickly as they arrive. I'm reminded of an inspiring saying from the recovery movement: "Begin with the truth and build on the firm foundation it provides."

 What has practicing yoga trained you for?

February 8

Accept that every journey is different.

After we practice yoga for a few weeks or months or even years, the fruit of wisdom starts taking root in our souls. We find the true guide within us that leads toward enlightenment. And we're never the same people again. Or not. It's completely possible that yoga will do absolutely nothing for your mind, body, or soul, and that's okay too. Friends of mine come to our studio and try out yoga all the time. And at least half of them never come back.

It's okay. There's no guilt, no judgments, no resentments, no pushy sales follow-up, and no awkwardness the next time we see each other. Part of my committed yoga practice is expressing acceptance for those who aren't as committed. It's not our job to convert, save, or fix others. Accept that they are on their own journey, and let them find their own way.

 Are you committed to accepting people's lack of commitment?

February 9

Find gratitude for everything.

Lying on the floor is a form of surrender and trust. When we finish the standing series and get down on our backs, teachers say to allow the floor to support us. That's harder than it sounds.

Sound like a ridiculous notion? Maybe for the first world. But there are tens of millions of people globally who don't have the luxury of that kind of trust. Some people live on floors that contain things that can harm them. Others live on floors that might crumble to pieces or get bombed out from under them. The smallest things that we take for granted are often immense gifts.

At our beautiful yoga studios, floors are clean and carpeted and level and safe. That's worth giving thanks for.

 Are you treating the ground that supports you with appreciation?

February 10

Big room, small crowd.

Practicing yoga mat-to-mat in a packed class creates an invigorating and communal energy, not unlike that of a church or a concert or a sporting event. It's truly magical.

But sometimes the most powerful and memorable yoga classes are the small ones—like when it's early in the morning after a big holiday or in bad weather and it's just you and the instructor and a few other people scattered about.

In a big room with a small crowd, it's your job to fill the space. You have to emanate your breath and energy and attention out toward each other. You have to work together to create the kind of heat and vitality and connection that make this practice such a joy. That's how you activate the power of community.

 When you walk into a room, how does it change?

February 11

Be flexible but not foolish.

Hot yoga has been clinically proven to increase flexibility. The higher temperature helps warm up the muscles, joints, and ligaments so that they're more effective with any type of stretching exercises.

On the other hand, according to rehab specialist Dr. Robert Gotlin, once you stretch a muscle beyond twenty percent of its resting length, you begin to damage it. Fair enough. There's a balance when it comes to flexibility.

Thankfully, those limits only apply to the physical realm. When it comes to our minds, it's not possible to be too flexible. That's what keeps me coming back every day. The heat allows me to access new flexibility in the room, which equips me to stretch beyond what I have done before outside of the room. So stretch your body and let your mind be blown. Not your knee.

 Do you believe you have to push yourself too far physically to reap the benefits of flexibility mentally?

February 12

Breathe your way back to joy.

Mentally disappearing can be an alluring and seductive activity. The danger comes when we do so at the expense of our present experience. Rather than be in the moment, we daydream or catastrophize through our existence.

Take yoga class. Sometimes I spend ninety sweaty minutes stressing and obsessing over the imagined details of some minor future event. This not only provokes anxiety, but also undermines any joy that might be had during class. I'm not present with myself. I'm alienated from my own body. And that keeps me from getting the most out of the moment.

Ever been there before? If so, here's a strategy to help you breathe your way back. Next time you notice yourself caught in a web of obsessive thoughts that block the flow of joy, try counting your breath. Four seconds on the inhale, two seconds on the pause, then eight seconds on the exhale. Literally counting it off in your head brings you back to the moment. Out of your mind, and into your body.

 How do you breathe your way back to joy?

February 13

Postures are palettes for the imagination.

The parallels between yoga and creativity are many and fascinating. Both are practices we use for physical, emotional, mental, and spiritual transformation. Both are canvases we use to express our highest selves. Poet Alan Shapiro's beautiful essay "Why I Write" states:

> Write for the pleasure of perfectly useless concentration. For the total immersion of the experience, the narrowing and intensification of focus to the right here, right now, the deep joy of bringing the entire soul to bear upon a single act of concentration.

Go back and reread that, substituting the word *yoga* for the word *write*. Still works. Because yoga, not unlike creativity, is one of those magical tools that enables flow. Looking from the outside in, you can never understand it. Standing on the inside looking out, you can never explain it. And that's a good thing. Some things in this world are best experienced, not explained.

 What other discipline does the practice of yoga parallel in your life?

February 14

Build a bias for action.

There are two main types of meditation: sitting meditation and moving meditation. The first approach uses *being*, i.e., stillness and concentration and contemplation, as the path to relaxation and enlightenment. Practices might include guided imagery, hypnosis, creative visualization, progressive muscle relaxation, and mindfulness breathing.

For people who have racing brains and hyperactive imaginations, that approach becomes frustrating and impractical. They'd prefer creating something over sitting around waiting. And so, moving meditation uses *doing*, i.e., activity and flow and momentum, as the path to relaxation and enlightenment.

Yoga is ideal for people who need physical movement to anchor themselves against their tumultuous waves of thought (or "monkey mind"). That's why I practice it, and it may be part of your rationale too. If you get frustrated by your inability to still your mind, maybe try moving your body mindfully instead.

 How are you developing your kinesthetic intelligence?

February 15

Build a foundation of resilience.

Yoga is tough. There's no doubt about it. It's tough on our bodies, tough on our minds, and if we practice with any kind of regularity, it's tough on our schedule. But the more we practice, the more we discover that yoga is also a fountain of resilience that keeps us afloat when times get tough.

With every pose we explore, we build up greater physical, emotional, and spiritual structures to put order into the chaos that our lives can become. Thinking back to all my many conflicts, injuries, workplace stresses, and relationship problems over the years, thank goodness yoga was there for me. Yoga allowed me to call upon whatever reserves of strength and faith were left to push through to the other side. Without it, who knows how poorly I might have handled those tough situations.

If you're in the hot room, feeling overheated and tired, struggling to balance your entire body weight on the tips of your pinky toes, remember this: Yoga is tough, but life is tougher. Train yourself to deal with the smaller irritations and challenges so that you're equipped for the larger ones.

 How are you building your ability to bounce back?

February 16

Build a practice that's truly your own.

"Stay on your own mat" is a helpful reminder to respect other people's privacy during yoga class; it's also a noble mantra that keeps us focused on our own practice, not someone else's. After all, each one of us has to put together our own path. What's best for our unique mind, body, and soul might be completely wrong for somebody else.

My wife, for example, likes to add in a few bonus stretches, crunches, and push-ups at the end of each class. It's how she winds down after a good practice. Whereas my ritual after class is to do a short mindfulness meditation, take a cold shower, and then make notes of all the ideas that came floating into my head.

We all do what works for us. And what works for someone else shouldn't keep us from using our own approach. It reminds me of songwriting, which has been the centerpiece of my creative life for more than twenty years. One of the lessons my music mentor taught me was this: *If you want to compete in clear air with your tunes, first you have to write all the pseudo-covers out of your system. Only then can you uncover your true voice as an artist.*

There's nothing wrong with getting inspiration from someone else's practice. Absolutely try different approaches to yoga until you find what fits. Try a diversity of yoga systems as you attempt to build a practice that's truly your own. But do stay focused on your own journey. Because there are just as many ways to do yoga as there are students to practice it.

 Are you keeping the focus on yourself?

February 17

Build momentum in your day.

Everybody needs a good on-ramp. A ritual that prompts a work mindset to start our day. A process that merges us into the real world and ensures that our days have a cadence and rhythm. A routine that gets us in the mood, in the flow, and in the zone so that by the time we actually hit the highway of life, we're traveling at the same speed as traffic, and can navigate the road effectively.

Early-morning classes are perfect for this. Not just for your own sanity, but for the sanity of the people you work with. Then again, everybody needs a good off-ramp too. Practices that merge from the workday back to the rest of life. Evening classes are perfect for that. Not just for you, but for your family too. Learn your rhythms, and honor what you need at different times.

 What's your on- and off-ramp?

February 18

Take down your defenses.

Humanistic psychologist Carl Rogers wrote that the biggest shift in his approach to therapy happened when he stopped thinking about how he could treat and cure his patients, and started wondering how he could provide a relationship that his patients could use for their own personal growth. It's a profoundly effective way to engage with people. Surrender the impulse to rush in and save the day and stand in awe at the emergence of the self.

I relearn this each time I practice next to a rookie student. The fixer in me wants to interrupt the beginner's practice and say, *Let me show you, here's exactly how you can do this pose right.* But that's not the point. People don't need prescriptions, they need relationships that serve as a secure base. A reliable source of emotional renewal, nourishment, safety, and security in the face of everyday challenges.

Once you stop trying to change people, they're able to see themselves more clearly. And from that place they can grow into the person they need to be.

 Are you curing people, or providing a relationship that they can use for their own personal growth?

February 19

Do the work.

When I was in college, I had lower back problems. It's kind of embarrassing when you're only nineteen and everybody expects you to be strong and flexible and resilient. But your body never lies to you. I remember my low point, literally and figuratively. It was just another night at our house the summer before junior year. One minute I was eating dinner with my family, the next I was incapacitated on the living room floor with horrible shooting lumbar pains that felt like an electric shock. The worst part was that my eighty-year-old grandfather had to run to the kitchen to fetch me an ice pack. Probably a sign that I needed to make a change.

My mom, a personal trainer, suggested that I start coming with her to the gym to stretch, strengthen my core muscles, and improve my overall posture. *Ugh. Sounded like work to me. No, thank you.* Instead, I opted for a deep tissue massage. Sixty bucks for sixty minutes, aromatherapy candles, relaxing music, and an attractive masseuse with strong hands? Felt like the right choice to me.

Treating the symptom always feels easy. Treating the source always feels like work. Often, we opt for the former. It's no wonder my back never healed. At least, not until years later, when I started practicing yoga. My mom was right. If we truly want to make a change that sticks, we ought to focus on the solution that involves actively working to improve our situation.

 Are you trying to take a shortcut to healing?

February 20

Stop and relax.

Classes on weeknights can be particularly stressful. Students have been pounding the pavement all day. Out and about, doing their work, managing their families, and meeting whatever other demands their schedules have imposed upon them.

You rush around all day long. The yoga studio is one of the few places where you can actually slow down. What a relief: Knowing that for the next sixty or ninety minutes, there's nowhere to rush, nothing to achieve, and nobody to beat.

When you enter the studio after a long day, be sure to change your pace. The yoga room is a refuge for lightness. It's a delete button for the outside world. A sanctuary where we can remember who we were before the world told us who we needed to be.

 Are you busy telling people how busy you are?

February 21

By taking action, we reduce the intensity of the problem.

When our yoga room is at full capacity, we practice mat-to-mat. It's awfully tight. Students have to be especially respectful of other people's space, property, and energy. Otherwise it can make for a distracted, frustrating, and claustrophobic class.

I was recently practicing within inches of another yogi, when it came time for a standing series. As usual, the instructor suggested that we stagger horizontally, so as not to fling sweat or accidentally clip the person next to us. But the woman to my left wasn't paying attention. She just stood there, hands on hips, chugging water. Her inaction was driving me crazy, to the point of anxiety and paralysis. In that moment, I could feel the controlling instinct inside of me welling up. I wanted to tap her on the shoulder and say, *just walk toward the mirror, lady. It's not that hard.*

How many times have we all been in that same position? Waiting around for somebody else to take the first step before we move? It happens every day. What keeps us stuck is the belief that someone else needs to change before we can move forward. That others should align with our implicit expectations, rearranging their existence around our requirements for happiness.

Unless we remind ourselves that people are not here to meet our expectations. Unless instead of making so many unbalanced, burdensome demands on others, we learn to take our own action. To readjust our own posture and position and move closer toward our goals, while granting others the space to do the same. It works in yoga, it works in business, it works in marriage and love, it works everywhere.

 What expectations do you have that lead to frustration?

February 22

Call upon the full range of your faculties.

At my yoga studio, our instructors remind us to use every part of our body to achieve the total expression of the posture. Even the parts that are relaxed. Just because something is disengaged doesn't mean it's unimportant, they say.

I've seen this principle play out during every class. It's the stillness of one leg that fuels the exertion of the other. It's the rock-solid locked knee that frees up the motion of the lumbar spine. Our relaxed, drama-free facial expression counteracts our inevitable muscle exhaustion. Every bit of ourselves serves a purpose.

 Are you making use of everything you are?

February 23

Calm down your mind, build up your space.

Taking a breath not only gives our mind calmness, it gives our body space. Paying keen attention to our inhalation and exhalation gives our body the physical stretch to reach just a little farther and hold the pose just a little longer.

For example, during *paschimottanasana*, or seated forward bend, our final stretching pose, we straighten our backs, hold our big toes with peace-sign fingers, and flex our feet to be parallel with the mirror. Every time we inhale, we elongate the spine a little bit more.

It's like magic. By progressively lengthening the breath, we find the body follows suit. The oxygen creates new space we didn't realize we had. This technique is especially impactful for those of us who have personal space and boundary issues. In those moments when we're feeling violated or restless and claustrophobic, all we have to do is take a breath. It doesn't just calm down our minds, it builds our capacity for going beyond our limits. There is always more left in the engine if we only breathe into it.

 How can your breathing produce calm?

February 24

Let your practice change.

I've been doing yoga for many years, long enough to have watched my experience evolve. In the beginning, my practice was largely physical. The purpose was to develop a healthier relationship with my breath and body. Next, my practice became highly spiritual. The purpose was to develop an existential connection.

Later, my practice became highly emotional. The purpose was to work through my feelings and problems. More recently, my practice has become highly communal. The purpose is to share my humanity with the other practitioners.

Whatever your reason for practicing, there's no right or wrong. Yoga is a mirror for what's going on in your life off the mat.

 How has the arc of your yoga story evolved?

February 25

See past your weaknesses.

When my various injuries flare up during yoga class, it makes me feel vulnerable, fragile, and scared. Not to mention frustrated, since my body won't allow me to perform some of my favorite postures, like camel and standing bow.

But that's not necessarily a bad thing. I'm reminded of an article published by one of the most renowned inpatient drug and alcohol rehab centers in the country. The therapists there tell patients that accepting their brokenness is the first step to a new kind of wholeness. Every aspect of the journey, including the difficult and seemingly unbearable moments, is essential to the final destination. Similarly, when you go to yoga class and start feeling varying degrees of twinges from your joints and muscles, accept and appreciate them. They are the doorways to your humanity.

 Can you see your limitations as more than obstacles?

February 26

Leave the yoga room (and world) better than you found it.

We say at my yoga studio that the first posture is getting there. It's not a joke. Ask anyone who's ever had to take public transit through two feet of snow to arrive on time for the sunrise class. Showing up is practically fifty percent of the work. But there is another invisible posture besides showing up that students often forget they're obligated to perform when class is finished. That's cleaning up after ourselves. Clearing the space. Wiping up the sweat we left behind and leaving the yoga campsite better than we found it.

It's an easy thing to forget, especially if you're trying to get to work on time. That's why we recently posted a new sign outside the door of our studio. It reads: *The Twenty-seventh Posture*, and it asks people to be respectful of their space and clean up after themselves and wipe down their rental mat before they leave.

You know, basic adult stuff. It takes less than a minute and saves the studio tons of time and frustration. Proving that if the first yoga posture is getting to the studio, the last one is leaving it better than we found it. After all, the word *posture* means not only the position of our limbs and the carriage of our body, but also our mental or spiritual attitude.

 Which invisible postures are part of your practice?

February 27

Invest in community and watch what happens.

I once visited a yoga studio that had a chalkboard above the front desk. The teacher wrote the names of all the new students for each class. And throughout the day, veteran students would leave encouraging comments or words of wisdom.

It not only made me feel welcomed, but also gave me a few helpful pointers about the postures. Imagine if every space made that kind of commitment to community. Perhaps you could start by doing something similar in your own life. Sometimes we forget our own power to impact others with the smallest gestures.

 How are you creating instant belonging?

February 28

Commit to stillness.

When it's a hundred degrees and sweat gushes out of every pore of your body for ninety minutes straight, it's kind of hard not to wipe, itch, scratch, pick, pull, or adjust something. The discomfort gets to us and makes us think we have to act to change it.

In those moments, remember that to practice perfect stillness amidst external stimuli is to be confronted with who you really are. That's when you can't hide from your truth. Sounds simple, but it's actually the most challenging part of class. Anyone can touch head to knee. But to just sit there and do nothing for sixty seconds? Especially when you might feel some physical discomfort arise? Yikes. Most people are so voluntarily overbooked and crazy busy that the mere thought of absolute stillness gives them an ulcer. They can't stand a moment of feeling an impulse without giving in to it.

But if you can practice stillness in the studio, you can practice stillness anywhere. Muscle memory is a beautiful thing. From stillness comes lucidity. And from lucidity comes the ability to listen to your intuition, no matter what distractions arise.

 How much time can you spend in stillness?

February 29

Put in the groundwork.

When I first started practicing hot yoga, my instructor gave me a valuable strategy for hydration. She said that if you wait until you're thirsty to reach for water, it's already too late. Hydration starts the night before. Don't come to class thirsty, or you'll be in a world of pain.

Her advice reminds me of the classic Zen Buddhist mantra *Dig your well before you're thirsty*. The concept has applications in almost every discipline. In business, if you're waiting for a company-wide survey to tell you what employees really think, it's already too late. In investing, if you're waiting for the market to tell you that a need exists, you've missed your window. In creativity, if you wait around until inspiration strikes, you'll never start.

Instead, start now, with one step.

 How do you dig your well before you're thirsty?

March 1

Confront the invisible posture.

The great twentieth-century thinker J. Krishnamurti wrote that every waking moment is another invitation to let go of the image of how life should be and embrace the moment as it actually is. Bowing to it, honoring its texture, shape, and taste, even if it's bitter. Taking what is given, receiving what life offers on the canvas of now.

It's an apt message for any yoga practice. Because each time we return to the mat, we're confronted with the invisible posture. The pose we never win awards for. It's the attitude of unconditional kindness toward whatever we may be experiencing.

If the body doesn't bend the way we expect it to, we let it go. If the water isn't as cold as we'd like, we let it go. If the yoga room is super crowded and we don't secure our usual spot right by the window where there's a nice little breeze, we let it go. If there's a huge, sweaty guy practicing next to us whose flop sweat accidentally drips right into our water bottle, we let it go.

The key is not making a problem out of not always getting what we want. Not letting it become our nature to always be demanding things as we wish them to be. That's our yoga for today. Focusing on the way life is, not the way it should be.

 How well do you let go of the image of how life should be?

March 2

Correct the habits that have limited us for so long.

Happiness is a mental habit. So is depression. Both of these emotional states result from our lifelong practices and patterns of conscious thought. We don't have to remain slaves to our routines. Cognitive behavioral psychology research indicates that any conditioned habit the human brain has learned can be unlearned. Even if we're predisposed to a particular behavior, we can still train ourselves to act otherwise.

Change takes time, patience, and forgiveness. Without those elements, we might never give our bodies and minds the necessary time to memorize the new habits we are starting. Author Gretchen Rubin's happiness research on the invisible architecture of everyday life offers a solid suggestion: Don't focus on rewards to motivate yourself. That undermines habit formation. Instead, she says, find your reward within the habit itself.

That was my challenge with yoga for many years. As a classic racing-brain creative, at first I found stillness to be torture for my mind. But with the help of my instructors, I learned to stop treating yoga as a tranquilizer, and started delighting in the daily practice. There was no finish line. All that mattered was enjoying the race.

Whatever habit you're trying to learn, or in most cases, *unlearn*, find your reward within the habit itself. Humans always assume things are going to be easier in the future. We think to ourselves, okay, starting tomorrow, I'm going to be perfect for the rest of my life. But changing habits takes real work. It also has real benefits.

 How are you learning to let go of what limits you?

March 3

Dare to be a beginner every day.

"It's never too late, it's never too bad, and you're never too old or too sick to start from scratch once again." That's the mantra of hot yoga that Bikram Choudhury has been saying for decades. Its meaning? That we are all potential novices. Interestingly, the word "discipline" comes from the word *discipulus*, which means student. This suggests a few things.

First: Declare your incompetence. Admit what you know you don't know.

Second: Learn to love mistakes. After all, a mistake ceases to become a mistake the moment you learn from it.

Third: Try not to be too hard on yourself. Let go of the self-criticisms that make discipline a big bite to swallow.

Fourth: Be patient. Every great chess player was once a beginner.

Remember, if the road to victory were smooth, everyone would already be there.

 Are you prepared to start from scratch?

March 4

Decide how much discomfort you can absorb.

Moving forward, establishing momentum, and executing our goals are all uncomfortable actions sometimes. But you can't expect to thrive only when things are safely within your comfortable grasp. Risk, struggle, and failed efforts are all necessary in order to make progress.

That's what drew me to yoga. You stretch yourself to the point where pain is a possibility, but not a reality. Each time, you may be able to go a little further into the posture. That awareness prepares you to handle future discomfort when it comes.

 What are you pretending not to be uncomfortable about?

March 5

Flex your mental toughness.

Anything that requires perseverance improves us. Even when we lose or when we see no visible signs of progress, we can't help but persevere. Doing hard things makes us better. As the motto of the Royal Air Force goes, *Per ardua ad astra*: Through struggle to the stars.

Yoga is an ideal way to build this very muscle. Not only does the practice help us improve our flexibility, strength, balance, endurance, and aerobic capacity, it also deepens our mental toughness. Every time we fall out of a posture and jump back in. Every time we show up on the mat when we're not in the mood. Every time we stay in the room when we feel the urge to run and hide. These moments of perseverance all improve us.

Maybe not in a way that makes us look sexier in our moisture-wicking high-tech yoga pants. But the very act of persisting signals our willingness and desire to show up for the struggle. And that's what really counts.

 Are you welcoming every opportunity to build your resilience?

March 6

Deepen your response flexibility.

Yoga teaches us flexibility of the body, but also flexibility in our responses to the world around us. The practice deepens our ability to pause in the face of a strong emotional stimulus, so that instead of reacting immediately as we normally would, we can pause for a split second and *choose* how to react. Viktor Frankl wisely called this moment "response flexibility." He said that between stimulus and response there is a space, and in that space lies our freedom and power to choose our response.

That's what yoga offers. Hundreds of those micro-spaces in which to deepen our response flexibility. To stop for a breath or two and acknowledge that our experience, positive, negative, or neutral, proves that we choose how we respond. It's like a latex therapy band for the soul.

 Are you as committed to putting an end to unhealthy responses as you are about touching your toes?

March 7

Practice the power of waiting.

All of the greatest yogis in history had a capacity for delayed gratification. That's what made it possible for them to achieve goals that most students would never tackle. They were willing to spend a whole year trying to bend their spine and execute the full expression of *one* posture.

"Gheranda's collection," one of the three classic texts of hatha yoga, says there are over eight million postures in total. Talk about delayed gratification. Are you that patient? Of course not. No mortal is. And that's our chance to *develop* patience.

We accept that if a yoga posture doesn't click right away, we should not consider the whole effort a failure. We believe that our body soaks up the benefits, even on our worst days. And we trust the ongoing effort of this practice, even when the results are not immediately evident.

 Are you prepared to start a practice that demands patience?

March 8

There is only the present moment.

In yoga there is no end point of completion, only continuation of the journey. There is no point at which you've "made it." There are no winners or losers. Filmmaker Richard Linklater said it best in his movie *Waking Life*: The ride does not require a destination, only occupants.

This mindset can transform your yoga experience forever. When you treat your whole practice as only a succession of nows, all of the anxiety and stress and expectation that once filled your mind floats away like a vapor trail. All that's left is you and your mat.

The same mindset can be applied to anything you do. When you celebrate the fact that you're here for the ride and let go of the need to actually get somewhere, the journey is that much more enjoyable. When you next lay down your mat, remember to bring your attention to the present moment.

 What is your yoga a metaphor for?

March 9

Accept your perfection.

The hardest part about being a new yoga student isn't compacting your body, it's comparing it. We look around at all these flexible, strong, sweaty bodies that look like wet noodles and think to ourselves, *Wow, my body will never look like that.* Maybe not, but by comparing ourselves to some unrealistic, nonexistent standard, we're always failing.

During a recent toe stand posture, my teacher made a comment to one of the first-time students. He said: *Your posture is perfect; it just looks different than everybody else's.*

It's perfect for you, where you are in your practice, right now. Tomorrow and next week and next year, it will still be perfect. Regardless of how different it looks from everybody else's. I wish somebody had told me that during my first class. Because one of the most common ways in which we imprison ourselves is through comparison.

 Is comparing yourself with others making you forget the uniqueness of your own journey?

March 10

Direct your attention in a more conscious manner.

I recently sustained a minor groin strain. Nothing that required official medical attention, just my own personal awareness during physical activities. It's uncomfortable at times, but the advantage is that having an injury forces me to practice yoga and walk through the world with more attention focused on that particular part of my body.

That keeps me present, makes me feel alive, and challenges me to engage other muscles I might otherwise ignore. Even our injuries have messages for us if we stop to listen.

 How might your injuries become a gift?

March 11

Don't disappear into logic.

People often struggle to be in touch with their emotional life because they process their issues intellectually, bypassing what they're actually feeling. We would rather step back from our feelings and analyze them, rather than allowing them to exist.

Sigmund Freud, the founder of psychoanalysis, explained that this intellectualization is a defense mechanism for avoiding anxiety. We attempt to think our way out of our feelings. We treat the situation as an interesting problem to solve, one that engages us on a cognitive basis, while the emotional aspects are ignored as being irrelevant.

That couldn't describe me more accurately. I'm the kind of person who always feels most at home inside his head. The process of intellectualizing is useful when it keeps us from reacting to life impulsively and irresponsibly, but only through complete emotional development are we offered the greatest degree of leverage in attaining our full potential.

That's one of the benefits of practicing yoga. When you're sitting in a hundred-degree room for ninety minutes straight, with nothing to do but stare in the mirror at your naked, sweaty body, intellectualization isn't an option. Trust me, I've tried. Yoga has a tendency to bring any and all emotions you've been storing inside your body to the surface. If I'm ever not sure what I'm feeling about something, I go into the studio and listen to my body. Unlike my mind, I know it will never lie to me. And anything that helps us create a healthier relationship with our emotional reality is a good thing.

 Are you treating your emotions as objects of contemplation, or opportunities to feel?

March 12

Openness is something you can arch into.

I love this mantra from one of my yoga instructors: *The shortest distance to the heart is through the body.* If there's an emotional experience you want to work through, you can back into it by changing your sheer physicality.

Take vulnerability. If you want to practice being seen as you truly are and allow yourself to be affected by the world around you, camel pose is the perfect posture. Not only is it the deepest backbend of the hatha series, it's also the only posture that fully exposes your throat, heart, belly, and reproductive organs, all at the same time. Doesn't get much more vulnerable than that.

I remember my first few months as a yogi. What I found was that the more I practiced, the more my body adapted. And after about a year, I finally bent my way to the full expression of camel pose. Interestingly, I also noticed greater vulnerability in other areas of my life. My openness to risk, uncertainty, and emotional exposure dramatically increased. As the body goes, so go the heart and mind.

 What might yoga open you to?

March 13

Reap dividends that are not found anywhere else.

Yoga gives us a strong physical base on which to stand, but also a strong spiritual base on which to expand. More and more with every posture we practice. The good news is that this experience has nothing to do with God, religion, faith, or theology, and everything to do with listening to and acting upon the mysterious messages within.

That's the divine source we've all been looking for. The best and highest version of ourselves. Sound hokey? Seem new-agey? Sure.

The more important questions are: Does it work? Does it help you evolve as a human? And will it transform you into a more compassionate and joyful person on and off the mat? As my instructor tells first-time students: Yoga is a practice that will pay us back in spiritual dividends that are not found anywhere else.

 When was the last time you got a swift, spiritual wake-up call that altered your reality forever?

March 14

Do you need this, or "have" to have this?

In my early years of practicing hot yoga, I developed a habit of bringing two frozen water bottles to my class. It was a bit excessive, but there were few things in the world that felt more refreshing. It was almost indulgent. Especially when the room was overly hot, humid, and crowded. The moment that icy water first touches your lips, you're whisked away to heaven like a sweaty, shirtless model in a soft drink commercial.

The only problem is, on days when you're running late and you forget to grab your frozen bottles, you show up to the yoga studio like a deprived toddler, pouting because he doesn't have his precious little ice pacifiers to get him through class. Meanwhile, there are almost eight hundred million people around the world who live without clean drinking water.

Lesson learned: Frozen water is an attachment. And every time we let go of our attachments, we move into another level. Use this framework to examine each item on your list of things that you think you "must have" to do your practice. One of my instructors challenges us on things like this by asking: *Do you need this, or "have" to have this?* Usually the latter.

 What's on your list of things you have to have to make it a good class?

March 15

Relax into discomfort.

Our teachers constantly remind us that it is possible to simultaneously experience comfort and discomfort. Sounds contradictory, but it's true. When you learn to respond instead of react, to breathe into that which makes you uncomfortable, you can move past it into another level of the posture. When straining to touch your forehead to your locked knee, you may discover a pocket of stillness that supports your stance. The exertion can lead you into relaxation.

What's exciting is that we eventually learn to apply that same principle out in the world. Yogis practice relaxing into discomfort during daily life. Slowly you start responding instead of reacting to what the world hurls at you, leaning into the feeling to find its lessons. That response paves the way to transformation.

 Are you at peace with discomfort?

March 16

Don't beat yourself up.

You will miss the mark from time to time. Learn to be okay with that. As my yoga instructor constantly reminds us: *Try not to pass judgment on yourself. When you interrupt stillness or fall out of posture, just notice it.*

Next time resistance gets the best of you and you drop the posture, don't be so hard on yourself. It happens. Learn from it, and keep moving.

 Will you be kind to yourself when you fall short?

March 17

Let your breath lead.

What do practicing yoga and brushing your teeth have in common? More than you think. During my latest routine checkup, my dentist gave an interesting direction: *Brush your teeth, don't scrub them.* When asked what the difference was, she said that most people brush way too hard. They assume frantic scrubbing back and forth will keep cavities away, when in fact, doing so can actually lead to enamel decay, sore gums, bleeding, and even teeth receding from the root.

Her advice reminded me of my yoga instructor, who often reminds students of a similar distinction: *Don't blow, breathe.* Same concept. When doing the postures, we assume that intense, dramatic breaths will somehow help us to power through the challenging poses.

But it's just the opposite. The yogi's goal is to draw slow, smooth, unremarkable breaths. To subtly nudge toward calm, not huff and puff and blow the house in.

 What kind of relationship do you have with your breath?

March 18

Find the right fit.

Joshua Liles, a close friend of mine who is also a brilliant yoga teacher, gave me this advice about yoga: *Find a teacher that won't let you fake it or force it.*

What an important balance to strike during class. All students should be pushed to their limits, their excuses and justifications for why they can't do things challenged in a loving, respectful, and helpful way. But they should never be pushed so far beyond their limits that pain or injury or danger is a possibility.

Fortunately, there are plenty of teachers to go around. In a 2016 study called *Yoga in America*, not only were there over fifty thousand registered yoga teachers nationwide, there were also two people interested in becoming a yoga teacher for every one current teacher. The resources are there. You can find the right instructor to meet you where you are and guide you to where you need to go. No settling necessary.

 What person in your life doesn't let you fake it or force it?

March 19

Let go of arbitrary goals.

How many calories do you burn while doing yoga? It's difficult to say. We all have our own metabolic baseline. It also depends on how hot the room is, how strict the teacher is, and how hard you work in the poses. Sometimes it's five hundred calories. Sometimes a thousand. Or, if you eat too much pizza for breakfast and need to lie down most of the class, the number is closer to zero. Perhaps a better question is: how much energy do you gain *after* doing yoga?

Even though the postures can seem tiring, they'll boost your system's adrenaline and fire you up. Not only that, but yoga requires you to focus on your breathing, which brings fresh, oxygenated blood to your muscles and brain.

Happens to me all the time. I arrive at class so tired that I can barely function, but afterwards I am bursting with energy and ready to take on the world. Try not to become too attached to some magic number of calories burned. Trust that your body is doing its work, and that yoga is gifting you what you need.

 How do you replenish your energy reserve?

March 20

Encourage and empower.

Equinoxes are regarded as the start of a new season. A chance to eliminate whatever is no longer serving you and make room for what will. Yesterday's developments are left behind, and new buds come up in their place.

Yoga works similarly. It's like spring cleaning: A chance to cleanse ourselves of feelings that we have processed, but no longer need.

Are you going through a change right now? Transitions are the perfect time to go deeper into your practice. Sweat out the old habits you're trying to let go of, literally create space in your body, and welcome the new to enter.

 How will you mark the new season?

March 21

Channel your flow.

The most valuable skill in yoga is learning how to concentrate. Mastering the ability to lock in at a moment's notice, anytime, anywhere, and get to work. That's what you notice about veteran practitioners. They have control over their psychic environment. And they take little time to bring their brain up to operating temperature.

Once they're locked into concentration mode, they don't ignore interruptions, they simply don't hear them. They don't swat off unproductive thoughts like fruit flies— they simply don't have them. And if you're on a tight deadline and the rest of the team is counting on you, being a master of concentration is priceless. High-wire artist Philippe Petit's brilliant memoir *Creativity* echoes this very sentiment:

> *Focus allows you to reach beyond your normal abilities. It cloaks your frequent intrusions into the domain of the impossible. But you must have a lifelong complicity with concentration. Otherwise the world cannot pour in freely.*

Do you have that level of control over your psychic environment? If not, here's a helpful exercise to deepen your ability to concentrate. What activity brings you into a state of "flow?" It could be running, writing, knitting, or playing guitar. How do you feel when you're immersed in that pursuit? Use that knowledge as a starting point for using that discipline in other areas of your life. Your ability to concentrate is stronger than you know. Maybe you're reaching for something that's already inside you.

 Why argue with the voice of distraction when you can train yourself not to hear it?

March 22

Don't just raise the bar, be raised by it.

Here's my favorite cheesy joke: *Two yogis walked into a bar. The third one used it to deepen their practice.* If you didn't laugh at that, you're probably not obsessed with yoga. Because that's how we oxygen junkies think. It's all part of the practice. Everything is grist for the yoga mill. Even the distractions and annoyance and injuries. They deepen us.

This mindset isn't limited to yoga. In her essay *The Getaway Car*, Ann Patchett's explanation of how and why she became a novelist takes a similar approach to the creative process. She says:

> *I am a compost heap, and everything I interact with, every experience I've had, gets shoveled onto the heap where it eventually mulches down, is digested and excreted by worms, and rots. And it's from that rich, dark humus, the combination of what you encountered, what you know and what you've forgotten, that ideas start to grow.*

Whether you're doing postures, writing books, or doing any other kind of creative work, make yourself entirely open to every shred of stimuli that crosses your path.

 Are you open to being changed by yoga?

March 23

Turn observation into action.

When our bodies speak, we must do more than take notes. We must take action. Because unlike the mind, the body is one of the few things in this world that will never lie to us. It may baffle us, but it will never bullshit us. We should think of and relate to our body as that good, caring friend whose feedback helps us learn about a part of ourselves that we need to discover. During a recent camel pose, my instructor led a short meditation that was truly empowering. He said:

> *Imagine a blue light shooting out of your throat. This vortex of energy governs communication, truthfulness, and expression. And so, whatever you want to say, whomever you want to say it to, know that you have the power to make your truth known.*

I literally felt the release in my body during that posture. When I came out of camel, I was floating. Interestingly enough, later that night I was able to have a difficult conversation with somebody close to me, voicing something that I originally planned on keeping to myself.

Lesson learned. Your body is your friend, and if you treat it with respect, it will support you in everything you need to do.

 Can you see your body as your friend rather than your enemy?

March 24

Avoid taking it personally.

Most of us have developed a hypersensitive relationship to the world. Unfortunately, that hypersensitivity results in our taking everything personally. We overanalyze, ruminate, and even become depressed and anxious over brief interpersonal interactions. I once spent an entire summer beating myself up over a one-line email from an angry reader. I became trapped in a bitter loop that left me awash in fury and resentment and made me feel irritable and on edge most of the time.

A woman I practice yoga with once gave me a great tip for this very situation. She said: Don't take things personally, because people are only talking about themselves. It's so true. Most people are just projecting their autobiography onto others. When we allow people's external criticism to trump our own belief in ourselves, the joke's on us.

Bikram reminds us that nothing external can steal happiness and peace away from us. If someone makes us angry, we are the losers. It's all about ownership: Refusing to give people you're not even invested in more power over you than they deserve or should be allowed to have. Remember, hypersensitivity can be an asset, but it's also a liability. Learn when to exert it, and learn when to holster it.

 Are you allowing the words and actions of others to define your reality?

March 25

Duality is the heartbeat of mastery.

In hot yoga, students experience the simultaneous practice of complete relaxation and absolute exertion. It sounds counterintuitive, but you can actually execute both actions in the same posture—as long as you know how to listen to your body. For example, standing bow posture practices an intense stretch of both arms in opposite directions. But it also requires that you relax your torso into your lower back while stretching.

That's the duality. Westerners aren't used to it, but it's a powerful muscle to strengthen. Not everything has to be black or white—sometimes, things can be both at once.

 What dualities do you need to honor in your life and business?

March 26

Let each asana strengthen your internal locus of control.

In yoga the body becomes an actor, not a reactor. It allows us to choose the qualities most important to us. Standing poses, for example, teach us confidence. Backbends teach us flexibility and openheartedness. Inversions teach us poise. Each asana, or posture, strengthens a different muscle.

A minute at a time on the mat, yoga takes us out of the victim position. We cultivate internal sources of power so that our action isn't dependent on our external environment. Ask anyone who's done yoga consistently for long stretches of time. Postures provide them with the opportunity to explore the self and observe how it reacts to life's many challenges and surprises. Yoga is a personal growth laboratory for working out in the body what we are working out in life. We can take control.

As the hamstrings go, so goes the rest of the world. At the end of our practice we feel more in control of our bodies, our minds, our spirits, and our lives.

 How has yoga affected your locus of control?

March 27

Embrace corrections as gifts.

There's no shame in being corrected. After all, yoga instructors are not trying to boss us around or embarrass us in front of the class. It's not personal—it's about maximizing benefits, staying safe, finding balance, getting alignment, and attaining healing.

When you're struggling in half moon pose and the teacher comes over and nudges your arms back behind your ears and it kind of hurts in a good way, be thankful. Because there's nothing more satisfying than hearing a correction, listening to it, understanding it, and then executing the adjustment properly to realize a deeper expression of the posture.

In my early years of doing yoga, I would become bashful when teachers called out my name during class. But now I embrace it as a compliment and a gift. An invitation to excel. Besides, I have a nametag tattooed on my chest. I'm kind of asking for it. Getting an adjustment in a posture isn't about being "corrected," it's about letting someone in and availing yourself of that person's wisdom. Corrections teach us to be humble, to appreciate the insights of others, and to grow from their feedback.

 What's the best correction you received last week?

March 28

Engage the pause that refreshes.

Yoga allows to us enlist the aid of the body's most powerful mechanism for personal change: *the breath.* Not because the physical act of inhaling and exhaling actually changes us into something different. But because breathing, this highly holy and healthy practice that combines awareness, mindfulness, kindness, and focused intention, creates the space we need to calmly address the parts of ourselves that might not be working.

From that place, we can make whatever changes are needed. In a modern world that has all but eliminated pauses, this is not an insignificant skill. Remembering how to breathe isn't a joke or a cliché. It's the best chance we have for getting better.

 Are you allowing yourself to press the pause button on life?

March 29

All battles are fought within.

Albert Camus wrote that peace was the only battle worth waging. This profound idea first appeared in an essay about the savagery of the atomic bomb. But keep in mind, Camus was also an existentialist philosopher. There's a deeper layer to his message about the battles we wage inside our heads—forewarning people that the fight for the *inner* landscape is equally as important as what happens in the material world.

Each of us is engaged in a lifelong struggle against our own nature. If we have any intention of making this world a better place, these are the battles we must attend to early and often.

Before any authentic transformation of the world can be achieved, there must be an ongoing inner practice in the minds, hearts, and souls of those who inhabit it. The secret is to acknowledge, celebrate, and share our victories. Allow ourselves to feel proud of every step we take forward—even the seemingly insignificant ones.

I recently hit a milestone in my yoga practice in terms of my ability to notice, classify, appreciate, sit with, and discharge my uncomfortable emotions during class. I still have a long way to go, but in the ongoing battle between me and the old me, real progress is finally being made. I'm learning to forgive my past broken self and be proud of the current one I see reflected back to me in the mirror. That's a victory. One that I take pride in achieving, because I know that in the long arc of my life, that milestone adds to the foundation that will allow me to contribute at a higher level.

 How are you waging peace in your inner battles?

March 30

Enjoy the amnesia of the asana.

In the same way that sleep is the best form of overnight therapy, yoga is a powerful tool for sitting with and moving through our bad moods. Ask anyone who's ever walked into the studio feeling crappy and walked out feeling like a million bucks. Yoga releases us from the grip of anger, sadness, bitterness, and rejection.

It's difficult to remain furious for very long when we practice. Our emotions are like weather patterns. They have a beginning, a middle, and an end. After ninety minutes in the heat, the sublime indifference of the space makes us forget what we were so upset about in the first place. That's why I would like to launch a new business: *Divorsana*. A hot yoga conflict mediation program to help couples peacefully navigate relationship struggles and end their marriages with grace. Our tagline would be "It's not the heat, it's the humility."

Kidding aside, yoga's creation of a space where no one wins or loses has a great lesson for all of us battling to win a fight for our ego's sake. In conflict, wisdom resembles a child's pose.

 What does yoga help you forget?

March 31

Engage in the right dialogue with yourself.

Our fingers are always pointed outward about what could be better. The room is too humid, the teacher isn't engaging enough, my shorts are a little too snug, the heating duct is blowing hot air directly on my face, the guy next to me is breathing like a bulldog on a treadmill, and so on. Of course, none of those things is wrong. They just are.

The challenge is accepting them, embracing them, and even using them to further our practice. I actually like it when there's something distracting going on in the yoga room. It challenges my ability to focus. It deepens the valuable skill of being able to concentrate, anytime, anywhere, no matter what annoying little thing is attempting to throw me off course.

 Are you trying to place blame elsewhere?

April 1

Ensure that your day has a cadence and rhythm.

Doing early-morning yoga is a series of small but significant victories. First, there's the victory of dragging your ass out of bed when the alarm goes off and it's still dark outside. Next, there's the victory of pulling yourself together to get out the front door on time. Then there's the victory of arriving at the studio itself, which is painfully out of your control because of weather, traffic, public transit, and many other untamable forces. At last there's the actual yoga class itself. Depending on the room, the heat, the instructor, your dehydrated body, and the girl next to you who's frantically checking email on her phone in-between postures, this can clock in at another dozen small victories.

But you're not done yet. As the sun starts to rise and the street noise begins to swell, you only have about seven minutes to hose yourself off before making the commute to work, where you will likely spend the next three hours sweating through your clothes.

It's only nine in the morning, and you have already achieved twenty-seven small victories. Well done, Grasshopper. That's the whole benefit of doing early-morning yoga. The rest of the day is downhill. It ensures that your day starts on a high note. Whatever challenges and stresses and conflicts you face afterwards, nothing seems that hard in comparison.

 How might you arrange your day so you become unstoppable?

April 2

Pay no attention to the noise around you.

Practice with distractions. This helps you remain calm in the midst of chaos. By doing so in smaller situations, you develop a deeper ability to walk your truth through the larger storms on the horizon.

My urban yoga studio has been a blessing for me in this respect. In any given class, I'll be confronted with parking lot car alarms blaring, smelly people dripping their sweat on my mat, and screaming children outside the window. If you can stay committed to your core during that hubbub, you can do anything.

 What practice arena will train you to walk your truth when the road gets rocky?

April 3

Every anxiety is another chance to inhale.

Yoga has doubled my tolerance. Thanks to my practice, when I experience moments of discomfort, waves of anxiety, even bona fide bouts of physical agony, I've trained myself to breathe through it.

It doesn't make the sensations go away, but it changes your relationship to the experience. Turns out, when you greet temporary suffering with a welcoming and thankful heart, you can use its momentum against itself to convert it into a meditation.

 When was the last time you gave thanks for your discomfort?

April 4

We are all connected by air.

Breathing is the first thing you do in most yoga classes. Physically, it warms up our bodies and stimulates blood circulation. Psychologically, it centers our hearts and minds through the fundamental tool of the breath. Communally, it gets all of the students singing from the same yoga hymnal. Most importantly in that regard, every breath we take makes us interdependent.

That's not an insignificant thing. Breath is life. It's what connects us to other humans, animals, plants, and other living things on this planet. No matter how much we love being alone, no matter how often we think we don't need other people, the fact that the average person takes about nine hundred breaths every hour proves otherwise.

We're only alone in this world if we choose to be. During the pranayama, or breath control, portion of your next yoga class, remember that every breath we take re-affirms our connection to our fellow humans, and to Earth itself, from its plants to its animals. We all rely on the same life-giving force to sustain us.

 What does breathing mean to you?

April 5

Every day your body is different.

The dance of yoga is about showing up and seeing what body we have today. Trusting that our body is not who we are, just what we are currently experiencing. Consider a typical week of classes:

Monday My neck was stiff from sleeping all weekend.

Tuesday My whole body was dehydrated from the stupid summer heat.

Wednesday My legs felt like tree trunks rooting themselves in the earth.

Thursday My left contact lens came out during camel pose.

Friday My digestive system was out of control from eating fat-free popcorn at work.

Saturday My sweat angel looked like an oversized bowtie.

Sunday My final savasana made me feel like an ice cube blissfully melting into the floor.

As our teachers say, every day your body is different. The yoga doesn't change, you do. Our task is to respect our bodies, not fight them. The workaholic approach was to wait until our bodies gave out and forced us to rest. We've all had times when we ignored our needs and imposed an artificial structure that didn't serve us. No more.

 How often have you ignored or denied your body's responses and pleas?

April 6

Live every moment as a new page in the story.

After years of making war against the way things are, I finally realized that life is a story that takes its time unraveling itself. All situations unfold regardless of how we feel about them, irrespective of our precious agendas.

Surrendering to this reality is actually quite liberating. It helps us believe that there is wisdom in the unfolding of events exactly as they are. It encourages us to align ourselves with those events as they are happening, in real time. And it asks us to trust that whatever we're gaining from this experience is perfect for our growth.

The problem is, this surrendered approach to life runs crosswise to the grain of modern culture. Most people aren't willing to carve out time for an emotional state that the rest of the world is suspicious of. Most people aren't willing to accept that everything is perfect exactly as it is. After all, we live in a hyper-impulsive, quick-fix culture. Patience isn't taught or rewarded. Humans have been primed for immediate gratification, and if we don't have to wait, we won't. If you like the idea of accepting the universe as it unfolds at your feet, be ready for resistance. Not just from yourself, but from the people around you. Don't let their expectations make you feel that your path is wrong.

 Are you still assuming things should be other than they are?

April 7

Every piece of information is not a crisis.

Humans aren't the only animals that think, but we're the only animals that routinely drive themselves crazy with their thinking. In our modern world, where information comes at us from every angle, faster than we can possibly handle, we treat every piece of information as a crisis. And when we fail to realize the consequences that repeated catastrophizing can have on our psyches, we drive ourselves into a negative mood, a bout of depression, or, worse yet, a full-blown panic attack.

That's why we need filters. One filter that's especially helpful is to reduce decision-making to a simple binary question. Here are a few examples I use:

> Is my life better with or without this?
>
> Does this make me money, or does it make me happy?
>
> Is what I'm doing right now consistent with my number one goal?
>
> Will this course of action simplify or complicate my daily existence?

Every day when I think about *not* doing yoga, the answer to these questions pushes me through. Even if I'm tired or sore or sick or stressed or have a barbeque hangover from the night before, the answer to whether to do yoga is Yes. I've used questions like these for so many years that they've become second nature. Internalized processes are the key to a strong practice. By thinking less, we end up doing more.

 Can you simplify your thinking to cut through the noise?

April 8

Go beyond the surface.

Yoga is an ancient discipline, but it's also a growth industry. According to multiple studies, approximately ten percent of the adults in this country report doing yoga every year. That's over twenty million people. No wonder classes have been so crowded lately. Yet what we discover after showing up on the mat for a few weeks is that everybody *does* yoga, but not everybody *practices* it.

Huge difference. *Practicing* is about deepening your postures, *doing* about achieving them. Ask those who return to the yoga mat on a daily basis. The best part of a daily yoga practice is the commitment to seek what is fresh, spontaneous, and interesting in the same place you looked for it yesterday. The experience of observing and connecting and surrendering and growing. Not just going through the motions. As my instructor loves to say right before we start beginning breathing: *Just show up and see what kind of body you have today.*

What's more, anything can be approached as a practice. In an essay that Mohsin Hamid wrote for *The New York Times Book Review* about writing fiction, he explained that it was, in many ways, like a religion. A daily practice, a way of life, a set of rituals, and an orientation toward the universe. Whether you're doing yoga or putting words on paper, the universal principle still remains. Show up every day. See what happens. Experience what you've done before anew.

 Are you doing things, or practicing them?

April 9

Join the collective.

Doing yoga alone just isn't the same. In my experience, the more students there are in attendance, the better the class experience. Practicing yoga in a group setting cultivates a strong, empowering, and motivating communal energy that simply can't be accessed when you are in your room listening to an audio recording or watching a video tutorial.

There's just something magical about the collective experience. Even though we're all focused on our own practice, the effect of everyone working together provides an amazing group energy that benefits all. It's like the room itself is alive and breathing.

We support those who struggle, we admire those who move through effortlessly. And every time something greater than us passes through our bodies, we all get to ride that wave. Surf's up.

 How does practicing yoga with others impact your postures?

April 10

Choose what's best for you today.

Like many things in life, yoga is as hard as we want it to be. That's the beauty of the practice. It meets us where we are. It invites us to engage the level of intensity that works best for our bodies.

If we're feeling especially strong and energetic one morning and want to go deep and long in every posture, that's awesome. That will be a tough class. On the other hand, if it's been a stressful day and we feel depleted and just want to lie in savasana in the back of the room until we start sawing logs, that class will feel like a cakewalk.

We always have a choice in life. Make the one that serves you most fully.

 Are you listening to the body you have today?

April 11

Assert your boundaries.

I recently stumbled across an interesting article from an old issue of *Yoga Journal*. The columnist, Stephan Bodian, was reflecting on the exposure of the sexual misdeeds of a prominent swami, reminding readers that surrendering to a teacher should never involve surrendering their personal integrity. No matter who's asking, we should never relinquish our right to say No.

It's a good reminder that we all have the power to make our own choices. In every class, we can protect our space from invasions, or we can give away that freedom and say Yes just because we want to be seen as nice or helpful or a good student. In yoga and elsewhere, there's a difference between giving up our attachments and giving up our rights. Standing strong against external demands requires a solid definition of healthy boundaries. We need a clear sense of our inalienable right as human beings to have control of our own bodies, feelings, and ideas.

 Are you able to hold a courageous conversation to reinforce your boundaries?

April 12

Step away from the guns.

Popular culture, mainstream media, and even ancient mythology have historically portrayed attractiveness, health, and power through images of strong, muscular, bulging arms. They are universally used as a symbol of physical prowess and desirability.

But although strong arms were certainly evolutionarily advantageous, they're not the only indicator of strength. My yoga instructor loves to remind us that our arms are merely accessories. The purpose of our practice is learning to rely on the muscles in our upper back, hips, chest, legs, shoulders, and core to support us, not just our bronzed biceps.

To that point, I once practiced yoga next to a professional bodybuilder. The guy was a monster. His arms looked like legs. Halfway through class, he collapsed into a pile of tears and pain due to a severe lower back injury and had to be carried off to the hospital. So much for arms being the universal symbol of health.

Each of us has his or her own assumptions, biases, misconceptions, and expectations about what we *think* success looks like. But just because something appears attractive in the mirror, on the balance sheet, in the marketplace, or on the screen, that doesn't guarantee its worth.

 Are you letting yourself be fooled by appearances?

April 13

Pobody's nerfect.

When you practice on a regular basis, the goal isn't to achieve perfect posture and absolute stillness and full expression in every single asana. The goal is to sweat your way into something interesting. To uncover a new understanding about your body, your breath, and your brain.

That's why our teachers call it yoga practice, not yoga perfect. When you fall out of posture, that's a good thing. Your muscles are learning something. Besides, this isn't a competition. It's not about winning and losing. Yoga, and life, are much bigger than that.

 What did you discover about yourself during your last yoga class?

April 14

Expect nothing and receive everything.

Chuck Spezzano's brilliant book *If It Hurts, It Isn't Love* makes the critical point that without expectations, anything can be a gift. But if we have a picture of how the world should be, our expectations tend to make us feel oppressed. The more we expect, the less we are able to receive and be satisfied.

The irony, Spezzano writes, is that the closer we get to this thing that we *think* will set us free, the more resistance we feel to having it, because of all the increasing demands we place on ourselves. Sound like a lot of work? It is.

Take it from someone who has an advanced degree in expectation. White-knuckling the world is bloody exhausting. What's more, people can smell it. That's what happens when all of our precious little hungers are clamoring for attention. We create a halo of desperation around ourselves. I've probably showed up for a hundred yoga classes, wanting to perform the postures so well I could scream. And yet, the classes never turned out the way I thought. When you want something too much, it's never there. Expect less, and you just may get more.

 Are you in danger of hugging something so much that you suffocate it?

April 15

Extend your arm.

A key difference between yoga and other forms of exercise is that in yoga you're not solely depending on your own abilities. Whereas going for a run on the open road at the crack of dawn involves you and nobody else, taking a class with fifteen other students led by an experienced and knowledgeable instructor taps into the wisdom of the group.

You can use the communal energy. You can learn from other people's mistakes. And best yet, you can get micro-posture corrections from teachers whose sole purpose is to help facilitate the poses for you. Plus, it's a nice break from going it alone all the time. Yoga assures that you don't have to do all the heavy lifting by yourself.

A younger, more naïve, and less mature version of myself wouldn't have been swayed by this argument. For someone like me, who rarely allowed himself to need anyone, joining the yoga community was an unexpected exercise in healthy social connection. The question is whether we're willing to extend ourselves, both in the posture and toward the other. A real yogi knows that turning toward others is a gift to ourselves.

 What can you choose to do to not feel lonely?

April 16

Facts are to be faced, not fought.

It's tempting to expect existence to obey our wishes. To demand that the universe has an obligation to make us happy and to feel that we deserve a world that reliably conforms to our wishes and desires. In this naïve prioritizing of *I wish it were* above *It is*, we only set ourselves up for disappointment, disillusionment, and resentment.

Once we stop approaching how things are as barriers to success and start embracing them as facts of life, we're free. At last we're accepting reality on reality's terms, choosing to walk through the world from a position of empowerment, as opposed to helplessness. It's a liberating moment. The mere *thought* that we no longer have to work so hard to eradicate everything we don't like from our life? Wow, it feels like a boulder off our shoulders.

Yoga is the ideal venue for practicing this freedom, because when our muscles cramp and tighten, the natural response is to fight it. As yoga reminds us, the best way to manage the pain is to merge with it instead. To slow down in the sea of surging sensations and become one with it. To love it, lean into it, laugh with it, and look at it while the feeling magically fades away.

It's a small moment in the grand scheme of things, but it's great practice in developing a healthier relationship with reality. Who knows? Once you master the process of merging with your pain on the yoga mat, there's no telling what kinds of larger challenges you might be able to handle in the outside world.

 What are you resisting?

April 17

Fast heart, slow lungs.

Hatha yoga breathing, which is smooth, continual, and consistent, does wonders for my racing brain syndrome and monkey mind. If you're not familiar with this experience, it's when your brain overwhelms your nervous system and causes anxiety, restlessness, and a host of other mental maladies.

Fortunately, thousands of yoga classes have trained my breath to remain regular in all situations. Breathwork has dramatically improved my ability to calm my mind on demand. The good news is that you don't need a decade of experience to reap the benefits. Just remember this mantra: *Fast heart, slow lungs.*

The first two words represent the many stressors and problems and accelerations of life. Everything that you do not command. The second two words represent the breath. The foundation. The one thing whereby, when you own it, nobody can steal your peace. These four words will change your life. Every single thing that is outside your control offers an invitation to remember what is in your control: the breath.

 How can breathwork reduce stress and anxiety?

April 18

Fear is a natural reaction to moving closer to the truth.

Yogi Berra was not only one of baseball's finest catchers, but also one of its funniest characters. He was well known for his impromptu pithy comments and seemingly unintentional witticisms, known as *Yogi-isms*. One of my favorites was: *If you don't have it, that's why you need it*. It's a true Yogi-ism in every sense of the word, and it applies equally to the work we do on the mat. My instructor repeats a variant of it all the time: *The posture you like the least is the one you need the most.*

If you're avoiding it, that's why you should do it. I vehemently avoided camel pose for the first eighteen months of practicing yoga. The vulnerability of that position was simply too intimidating for me, both physically and emotionally.

Every time I sat out during that posture, part of me wondered if I was closing myself off from a whole universe of benefits. Maybe the scary posture was a mirror into my relationship with myself. Thankfully, I had great teachers and fellow students whose loving encouragement slowly stripped away my avoidance. They inspired me to banish the fears that undermined my courage. Ten years later, camel posture is the one I most look forward to in every class, its vulnerability no longer a threat to me.

Whatever it is that you're currently avoiding, Yogi Berra was right. If you don't have it, that's why you need it. Trust that you are ready to receive the gifts within what you're afraid of.

 Are you sweeping necessary changes under the rug in an attempt to avoid conflict with yourself?

April 19

Feeling better by getting better at feeling.

A psychologist friend of mine has a brilliant mantra for her patients: *You don't go to therapy to feel better, you go to therapy to get better at feeling.* If you ask anyone who's sat on a shrink's couch, it's absolutely true. Having a skilled, empathetic professional who asks you questions about your emotional state, and then actually listens, is an invaluable tool for healing. The therapist isn't solving your problems for you, but just giving you space to figure them out yourself.

Yoga works in a similar way. In fact, it's the best of both worlds. Because when you spend ninety focused minutes tuning into your body and confronting your truth in the mirror, you walk out of the room feeling not only better, but also better at feeling.

My yoga practice has deepened my emotional development more than any endeavor I have ever pursued. Nothing against my therapist, but my yoga studio has been the single most useful training ground for noticing and naming my feelings. No wonder there are so many shirts and stickers that read: Yoga is cheaper than therapy.

 Are you using yoga to its fullest extent?

April 20

Find a filter to process your experiences.

My yoga practice isn't just a great physical workout, it's also a venue for working through my emotions. Maybe it's because the room is a hundred degrees, but after a few postures, any feelings and emotions and inner struggles that needed to be dealt with, simply are. Not something to fight against or hate myself for. No "shoulds" have to be uttered in the hot room. It's a place where I can become a vessel for the Now and leave my anxieties and feelings to one side. We cling tightly to these, but the postures know better.

 Do you have a familiar place you go when you need to make sense of the world?

April 21

Find and develop your own internal supply of peace.

Reaching for an unhealthy coping mechanism like shopping, eating, or gambling is rarely necessary, often expensive, and almost never what we really need to get better. Most of the time, it just keeps us stuck in a cloudy fog of denial. And, in my case, a set of orange fingers from my favorite savory snack.

The goal, instead of trying to eat or drink or shop away our feelings, is to stop and deal with what's going on inside, right now. This is a very difficult habit to get into. The good news is that any conditioned habit that our brain has learned can also be unlearned. Sometimes we just have to enter through the side door.

Psychoanalyst Carl Jung's insights into tuning into the body's wisdom come to mind. Jung said that the hands often would solve a mystery that the intellect struggled with in vain. That's why yoga has become my number one diagnostic tool. It forces me to confront the whole self. And now, thanks to that daily practice, there are no longer any overwhelming feelings that I don't have a healthy coping mechanism for.

Think about the last time you got a professional massage. The therapist's hands are like flashlights in a darkened room. Where we're touched is where our attention goes, and that provides information we were not previously aware of. We may not even realize that we're tense or sore until we're massaged in our calf, neck, shoulder, or lower back. That physical experience gives us new information, which gives us new choices, which gives us the power to deal with whatever life hurls at us.

 How will you use the power of the body to access the needs of the heart?

April 22

Firm both of your bottom lines.

Yoga is healthy for your mind, body, and soul. It's also healthy for your company's bottom line. Aetna, one of the largest health insurers in the country, recently started offering free yoga classes to its employees. Over a fourth of their fifty-thousand-person workforce has participated in at least one yoga class. The reported results were fascinating:

A twenty-eight percent reduction in stress levels.

A twenty percent improvement in sleep quality.

A nineteen percent reduction in pain.

An average of sixty-two minutes per week of productivity gained.

Of course, this isn't the only example of yoga being used by an organization. More and more companies and communities and even correctional facilities are starting to awaken, both professionally and personally, to the many benefits of doing yoga. Although yoga might not be the panacea for our society's many problems, it's certainly one step in the right direction.

 How are you using yoga to enhance the rest of your life?

April 23

First you do yoga, then yoga does you.

When I wrote my first book more than seventeen years ago, my mentor said something I'll never forget: First you write the book, then the book writes you.

He was right. The process, production, and promotion of your art has a ripple effect that affects you forever, often in ways that you can't predict. Yoga, as a practice, works the same way. You don't just do yoga, yoga does you. That's the divine reciprocation of the practice.

For me personally, not only my body, but also my way of being, began to shift when I started to practice. Yoga helped me tap into a deeper part of myself. I may have started out trying to be in control of the postures, but soon I let them take the lead. That's when you really start to learn the lessons yoga has to teach.

 Are you allowing yoga to have its way with you?

April 24

Open yourself to love.

The Sufi poet Rumi said that it is not our task to seek love, but to seek and find all the barriers within ourselves that we have built against it. Yoga knocks out those barriers for me. Because the mirrors don't lie. They force me to confront even the most unlovable parts of myself and own them as part of my truth.

Without this practice, I could easily take all the shameful and noxious parts of myself and stuff them in a bag and decide that they're not lovable. But not anymore. Now that I've committed to showing up in the hot room every day, there's no way out. The barriers rise up in the practice, and can be dismantled one by one.

Slowly the walls I've built against loving myself have melted away. Quite literally, since the room is a breezy one hundred and five degrees. As a result I now believe that I'm blessed by the ability to receive love through many channels, including from myself, despite my imperfections.

 How can you seek love in your practice?

April 25

Focus on the postures, not on posturing.

A pastor friend of mine has a theory on communication. He says there are two ways to listen to people: We can perform, or we can participate.

Creating theatrical moments and scrambling to deliver the perfect nugget of inspiration so you can change somebody's world view forever—that's performance. Ever been on the receiving end of that codependent cocktail? Sounds like my twenties.

The other approach to communicating is participation. In this zone we organically engage with another person through curiosity and wonderment, not because we're trying to prove what we have to offer. Doesn't that sound like a healthier way to be?

It reminds me of yoga class. Some students show up to do the poses; others just show up to pose. The former couldn't care less about their hair or their costume or their location in the room or what kind of water bottle they're using. They just want to engage in their practice. But those who come to pose and put on a show are less concerned with doing the postures than they are with posturing. Make sure performance isn't sneaking into your own routine.

 Are you performing or participating?

April 26

Force yourself to flex your forgiveness muscle.

Each class is filled with small opportunities for us to choose forgiveness. We forgive first-timers for not following proper yoga etiquette. We forgive our bodies for not bending in the way we want them to. We forgive our minds for getting stuck on the mental hamster wheel. We forgive our hearts for judging the person in front of us. We forgive our instructors for accidentally dripping sweat onto our mat.

The list of forgiveness opportunities is infinite. Forgiveness is not something that we will ever be done with. But each instance counts. Each time we practice compassion for self and others, yoga is working.

 Have you stopped punishing yourself for what you think you've done wrong?

April 27

Free yourself from the anxiety of having to be in control.

Sometimes you do everything right, and it's still not enough. It's maddening. Learn to let go of trying to check all the boxes, however, and liberation awaits. Once you realize that control is an illusion and that the outcome of most situations isn't based on how much effort you exert, you can finally let go and let the joy carry you.

I meditate on this principle each time I practice. Especially when I have an injury. Whether it's a muscle strain, tendinitis, or lumbar pain, my brain gets angry at my body for being unable to perform every posture in the series. This brings to the surface one of my deepest fears, which is that I'm not as healthy as I think I am. Of course, that's just another ego delusion—the story I choose to believe about myself.

That's why I started accepting the reality of my body and freeing myself from the anxiety of perfection. Even if that means skipping my favorite posture every day for three months. What I found was that you can actually accomplish more with the energy of acceptance than the energy of control.

Keep in mind, surrender is not resignation. You're not waving a white flag and collapsing into complacency. You're just relieving yourself of the enormous burden of ruling the universe. Next time you fail to make headway in your endeavors despite working hard, allow yourself to feel frustrated. But only for a short while. Feeling sorry for yourself wastes a lot of mental energy. For now, try moving through the anger to discover the freedom waiting on the other side.

 In what situations do you have difficulty accepting yourself?

April 28

Say no to the drug of progress.

Peter Block, in *An Other Kingdom,* offers an inspiring narrative on community building. His vision of our future calls for an end to competition, scarcity, and efforts at endless improvement, and the beginning of abundance, fallibility, and infinite mystery. One of the action items in his philosophy is to kick our cultural addiction to the erroneous notion of progress. He writes:

> *We must put an end to the belief that a community or an institution or even a business has to grow or die to survive and have a meaningful life. Believing in enough means we can finally stop identifying with progress as the sole path to the good life.*

I've been saying the same thing for years. Contrary to popular conditioning, there are more important things in life than getting bigger and better and faster and stronger and richer. There's nothing wrong with wanting to make things better. But fetishizing efficiency, worshipping at the altar of productivity—these cravings only rob us of the capacity for joy and cause us to wonder what makes life worth living in the first place.

I notice this tendency often plays out in the locker room at my yoga studio. A new student will strike up a conversation with me. Inevitably, he will ask: *how long have you been practicing,* and *have you seen improvements?* To which I reply, *many years,* and *who cares?* Frankly, I'm not interested in getting better. I just love the practice.

 Is your romance with the progress of life preventing you from enjoying it?

April 29

Gain jurisdiction over your body.

Balancing stick (known as warrior three in some yogic traditions) is my favorite posture. It's invigorating, it's challenging, and it engages every part of your body and mind. From the side, your body looks like the letter *T*. You charge your legs and arms in opposite directions and hold the pose for the longest ten seconds of your life. The hard part is keeping your hips level and parallel to the floor. If you watch closely, most students unintentionally allow their hips to flare sideways, which throws off their balance.

It's frustrating as hell. Moving your hip is harder than it sounds. It's not a part of the body over which most people typically have control. In fact, my balancing-stick pose was wobbly for years—until a teacher gave me the following correction. She said: *Instead of trying to lower your hip down, point your foot back. Breathe into the deep stretch over the backside of your balancing leg, and your hip will move parallel to the floor naturally.*

The first time I tried it was like magic. Suddenly I had jurisdiction over a part of my body that always felt ungovernable. It's proof that many of our goals are accomplished incidentally, not intentionally. Once we figure out how to knock down that lead domino, everything in its path gets accomplished as a matter of course.

 Are you trying to lower your hip, when you simply need to point your foot?

April 30

Find gentle opportunities to observe possible flaws in your own thinking.

Mark Lundholm is a former criminal, mental patient, and homeless alcoholic who now uses stand-up comedy to help addicts thrive in recovery. One of his best-known mantras is *first thought wrong.* It is particularly pertinent for individuals suffering with the disease of addiction and their impulsive mindset, but it applies to us all.

The theory is that recovery is not the absence of bad thinking, but rather the ability to navigate through it with grace. If addicts follow their first thought, it will get them into trouble. But if they learn to take notice, take pause, and take alternative action, they can move toward healthier living. Even if it takes them an hour or a day or a week to get to the thought that's right, the addict's first thought, properly filtered, can eventually become the next right thing.

What I love about yoga practice is that it's all about forgiveness. It's about not beating yourself up for *having* impulsive thoughts, but simply *noticing* that you're having them, and then trusting that in the sacred space between, you can locate the healthier ones. What's more, it isn't exclusive to addicts. Every yoga student on the planet could use more gentle opportunities to observe possible flaws in their own thinking. As my instructor once said, any time a person takes the opportunity to let go of impulsive and unhealthy thoughts, that's yoga.

 What's your mantra for navigating through your thoughts with grace?

May 1

Use gentleness.

Our instructors not only give us valuable posture corrections, they also model how to give them correctly. It's a skill that takes years of practice and hundreds of classes to master. In fact, many new teachers are trained *not* to give corrections for the first six months of their career. It's not because they're lazy, but because they need to find their own energy before giving it back to students.

The teachers at my studio use a combination of compassion and confrontation in their corrections. They don't make us feel embarrassed about being human; they might even make us smile during the process. Best yet, if they notice that we have let ourselves slip back into old habits, like bending our knees on the setup of bow pose, or pitching forward on the exit of an awkward pose, they gently correct our course without making us feel that we have failed.

It's good inspiration for our own inner work, too. Outside of the studio, when our teachers are nowhere in sight, we must master the art of correcting ourselves with the same level of grace.

 What's the best correction you've ever received during a yoga class?

May 2

Get friendly with your neighbor.

My first few years of yoga took place in the Midwest. The studios were large, spacious, and sparkling clean, and you never practiced closer than two feet away from another student. When my wife and I relocated to a major metropolitan city, classes were different. Manhattan isn't what you would call spacious. I'll never forget our first class in our new neighborhood. We'd been in town two days. It was cold and snowy and blustery outside, and there were enough students crammed into the room to make the fire marshal nervous. Right before the stroke of eight, our instructor said: *Okay, folks, looks like we have to work mat-to-mat tonight, so get friendly with your neighbor.*

You should have seen the look on our faces. Our personal space vanished into thin air right before our eyes. At which point our instructor bent down and whispered, *Welcome to New York.* It was a rude awakening, no doubt. But also a perfect introduction to our new surroundings and an apt metaphor for living in a big city. When everyone's in your face, you can't escape—you can only engage with them. It's proximity-enforced acceptance. There's not enough time or space for judgment to enter.

As awkward and suffocating as it feels at first, ultimately, it's a good thing. Any time we can short-circuit our fear system and launch right into acceptance, our posture changes in every sense of the word.

 How many people did you go out of your way to avoid last week?

May 3

Get present with your physicality.

Headstands are hard. Doing the standing splits is hard. Balancing our body weight on our big toe is hard. Twisting our spine into a pretzel is hard. But that's not what scares us about doing yoga. What scares us is the *emotional* posture of the practice. Because no matter what style of yoga we try, and no matter what type of teacher we have, the challenge is the same: Somebody is going to suggest a new way of operating that goes against our preconceived ideas.

Now that's hard. For me, it required becoming *bodysmart*, as my teacher called it. Fighting the urge to disappear down the rabbit hole of my mind and getting present with my physicality. Letting my thoughts come and go like weather patterns and listening to what my muscles and joints and bones were telling me.

Talk about a new way of operating! It was a challenge. Still *is* a challenge, more than ten years later. But exploring your relationship to your body will allow you to attain heights greater than you thought possible.

 What practice helps you get present with your physicality?

May 4

Give compliments that matter.

The first time I attended a posture clinic, my body did things I thought only circus performers could do. Since then, my practice has never been the same. Afterwards I remember thinking, *how can I show gratitude for this accomplishment?* So after class, I approached our guest instructor with the following compliment: I thanked him for giving me permission to impress myself. He was speechless, and so was I. It was a moment we'd never forget.

Sadly, several months later I found out that the teacher had passed away. Apparently he was extremely sick with a terminal disease, even though none of his students could tell. All the more reason to give compliments that matter: You never know when, or if, you're going to see that person again. May as well leave them feeling essential to the world.

 Where can you be more generous in your gratitude?

May 5

Prepare for surprises.

The hard thing about hot yoga isn't the heat itself, it's what the heat brings to the surface. Both physically and emotionally, every class results in stuff coming up that we're not necessarily happy about, prepared for, or comfortable with.

Out of our bodies come sweat, cramps, tears, farts, and God knows what other biological surprises. And out of our hearts and minds, there's a stream of thoughts we'd prefer not to face. Wow. Sign me up for an unlimited yoga package.

But here's the secret to a strong practice. Whatever surfaces, our job isn't to judge or deny or flee or make ourselves feel guilty about it. Only to notice it. To observe what surfaces and say, *well, so there that is.* Then, move on with the posture.

 Can you simply be aware of what is, without giving it names and judging it for existing?

May 6

Would you rather be good *at* something or good *to* someone?

If you're the kind of person who hates losing and can't stand being bad at things, or who pretends everything can be fixed by working harder, yoga is going to be a struggle for you. As my teacher often reminds new students, you're not here to be good *at* something; you're here to be good *to* someone.

Namely, yourself. That's the true practice of yoga. Seeing how kind, loving, compassionate, and accepting you can be toward your own body, mind, and spirit. It's one of the few activities that not only isn't a battle to be won, but isn't worth the time and energy to fight.

Show up. Breathe. Listen to your body. Repeat. Yoga is like art. It doesn't have to be done well; it just has to be yours.

 How compassionate are you with yourself?

May 7

Exercise, or exorcise?

There's no hiding in hot yoga. Whatever emotions we've buried beneath the surface eventually have to come out. That's one of the reasons I sometimes cry sporadically in the middle of class. *What the hell? Where did these feelings come from?*

It's not that I'm responding to something that has actually happened to me, it's that the heat and humidity and intensity of the yoga unearthed some emotion I was trying not to feel. Despite my avoidance, it needed to be released.

Perhaps that's the best answer to the question *"Is doing yoga a good form of exercise?"* Yes. And it's also a good form of exorcise.

 What are you still afraid to feel?

May 8

Find your match.

For me, hot yoga wasn't love at first sight, it was *impact* at first sight. By the time I returned home after my first class, the only thought running through my mind was, *Wow, that was the hardest thing I have ever done in my life. When's the next class?*

That's how alive yoga made me feel. I slept the sleep of the just that night. Because this new practice wasn't merely a story inside my head, it was real-world application inside my body.

It's similar to how our approach to dating changes as we mature. Instead of the usual infatuation, addiction, and codependency that governed my past relationships when I was younger, yoga was based on good old-fashioned healthy compatibility. Yoga and I were simply good fits for each other. Make sure you're filling your life with things that have value for the long haul, not just initial surface appeal.

 What kind of relationship do you have with your practice?

May 9

Don't let yourself believe in invincibility.

When you're a workaholic, somehow all the warnings in the world don't quite convince you that it's time to stop. We have a preconceived narrative we cling to. We love to tell the lie that there's nothing wrong with putting in consecutive fourteen-hour days if we love the work and it feels like a calling and we're making a meaningful difference in the world. That we may as well just keep pushing until our body gives out and forces us to rest and take care of it. Then we can stop, but not before.

If that's the case, we're most likely running on the steam of a delusion. Convincing ourselves that our compulsions are serving something other than our own ego. It reminds me of something my yoga instructor, Carol, once said in regard to dehydration: *Don't try to be a soldier when your body needs you to be a saint.*

If you have to stop, rest, sit out, take a break, refill your water, go to the bathroom, or even lie down and sleep for the remainder of class, do it. Listen to your body, not your ego. Our daily practice should always allow unscheduled time for unexpected self-care. Time to listen to what our body needs, regardless of what our ego wants.

In short, we have to stop trying to impress ourselves all the time. Life is not a performance. There is no studio audience. There are no panel judges with numbered signs to score us. And taking a breather is just fine when needed.

 Are you still gripped by a mad delusion of invincibility?

May 10

Grow in your willingness to try things.

Yoga is more of a gamble than a guarantee. There is no way to know if we will enjoy the practice or even receive benefits from doing it.

But at the very least, we will grow in our willingness to try things. We may find that the minute we insert the key of willingness in the lock, the latch of possibility springs open.

Yoga was never something I saw myself doing—until I tried it. And then it transformed my life in multiple ways. Now the thought running through my head is, *I wonder what else I might try.* Because you never know. There might be another beautiful world waiting for you to step into it.

 Are you giving yourself an excuse to not try things?

May 11

A smile in the mind, a shift in the body.

My favorite yoga teachers are the ones whose words snap me out of my head and into my body. Here are a few of their most memorable commands from over the years:

Your ankle feels like an avocado pit inside your palm. Squeeze your butt cheeks tight enough to hold a dollar bill. Hinge your torso against your thighs like a grilled cheese sandwich. Point your hands toward the mirror like the pistol of a government spy. Hover over the mat like you're peeing in a Port Authority bathroom.

Each line is more ridiculous than the next, but that's their beauty. These silly but helpful words create a smile in the mind, which causes a change in the body. Each expression becomes a bell of awareness that chimes through our practice and makes us better.

 What's the funniest thing you've ever heard your instructor say?

May 12

Help reduce the risk of cognitive strain.

I have a tendency to intellectualize and overthink things. Using my rational mind to regulate emotions and solve problems is a useful approach for strategizing projects and getting things done. But when it comes to more interpersonal and relational matters, taking the elevator to the top floor and getting stuck inside my head isn't particularly helpful.

I've had to teach myself to go perpendicular and take leave of my mind. To create something more useful for the brain to do. Standing in a hot room for ninety minutes is perfect. Because it's too hot and too intense to think, which reduces the risk of cognitive strain. Once class is done, my head is as clear as a cloudless sky.

Having a wide repertoire of meaningful tasks at our disposal, should we get stuck inside our heads again, is the secret to giving our brains a break. Sometimes going over the same questions ad nauseam only keeps us stuck, and we need to know how to change the channel.

 How do you moderate your intellectual tendency to overthink?

May 13

Hold hands, not grudges.

I've never been one to hold grudges. Getting mad at people for making mistakes is exhausting. It's easier to let others off the hook and accept imperfect humanity, rather than wrapping myself up in righteousness and prosecuting people for crimes past.

But although I'm quick to let the actions of others roll off my back, I *do* have a tendency to hold grudges with myself. It's just my personality. I set unrealistically high standards for myself and get upset when I fail to meet them. The good news is, there are physical keys to help unlock the emotional doors that otherwise doom me to self-castigation. When there's a challenging emotional experience you want to work through, try backing into it by changing your sheer physicality. To repeat an instructor's mantra, the shortest distance to the heart is through the body.

Just ask the masters of yoga. They believe that the inability to forgive yourself stems from an imbalance in the heart chakra. This center of spiritual power governs the rib cage, lungs, diaphragm, and, of course, the heart. That's why students simultaneously love and fear poses like cobra, triangle, and camel. Because doing so opens the chest cavity and exposes vital organs. Doing so requires deep courage and vulnerability.

As the body goes, so goes the heart. That's why, for people who hold grudges against themselves, those postures are always worth the cost. They keep the positive energy flowing. They literally open your heart, which creates the necessary space to love yourself. Sure beats paying the price for your mistakes over and over again.

 What prevents you from asking for and receiving forgiveness from yourself?

May 14

‚ 9)

Time to ground down.

When we're feeling a bit wobbly in a standing pose the best move isn't to grip down with tight, anxious feet. My instructor reminds us instead to turn our feet into tripods, using the three corners of the foot (the big toe, the pinky toe, and the center of the heel) to ground into the support of the floor beneath us. That means releasing the points of our feet that aren't touching down instead of keeping them tightly clenched. Grounding down is a tool for equalizing the pressure and building greater foot and leg strength. To the point that we could practice yoga on a sheet of ice if we needed to.

Taoist mystics have actually been preaching the message of grounding down for years. As the ancient scripture goes, *he who grips at nothing therefore loses nothing.* When we hold on instead, clutching and clinging too tightly, we receive the rope burns of attachment. Not only that, our foundation suffers.

What are you still afraid to let go of? Perhaps it's your mat or towel or ice-cold water or favorite spot in the yoga room by the window. Whatever it is, it's time to ungrip. That's the real yoga. Learning to release our clamp of control on life and trusting that our foundation will support us.

 Where in your life are you gripping too tightly?

May 15

Emphasize respectfulness.

In any given yoga class, every act says something about how we regard or honor ourselves, and how we regard the people and things around us.

If we consciously choose a spot on the floor that gives the students behind us a clear line of sight to the mirror, that says something. If we arrive two minutes before every class and make a ruckus as we enter in the middle of the first posture, that says something. If we lead the round of applause for newcomers and first-timers who slogged through their first class, that says something. If we produce a sweat angel the size of a small freshwater pond and neglect to mop it up before we leave, that says something too.

If we greet everyone in the locker room regardless of familiarity and seniority, if we complain to the instructor that the room temperature is not to our liking and start moving around until we find the perfect spot, if we spend a disproportionate amount of time during class staring at the people around us like they're lunch, it all says something. Make sure what you're communicating with your actions is in line with your values.

 What do people think when they hear your life speak?

May 16

Resist panic.

Renowned creative thinking expert Edward de Bono's research on lateral thinking discovered that in hotel fires, more people were killed as a result of panic reactions than by the fire itself. It's a frightening fact, and a reminder that we are our own biggest threat. Even in the midst of a crisis, when the world is burning around us, the thing that is most likely to destroy us is our own inability to react intelligently.

Few of us ever find ourselves in the middle of a hotel fire, but that doesn't mean we shouldn't work to improve our *response flexibility*, meaning the ability to pause before we act. My yoga instructor constantly tells students to do this when the room gets especially hot. Before you reach for water, before you flop down on your mat, before you walk out of the room, she says, try breathing through it. Don't buy the story the mind is selling. Just breathe.

Dum spiro spero: Where there's breath, there's hope. Nine times out of ten, it works. Despite room temperature or muscle soreness or physical exhaustion, a calm, ten-second breath is surprisingly effective. Learn to resist a panic reaction to the surrounding fire. Because in between stimulus and response, there is a space for an intelligent choice.

 What's your healthiest response to crisis?

May 17

Loosen your relationship with the future.

It's the truest natural law of the universe: The more we expect, the less we receive. Here's a helpful quiz to find out just how addicted to expectation you really are:

Do you control situations so that they can come out the way you want?

Do you try to force the direction your life should take?

Do you get trapped in thoughts about what should be coming to you?

Do you like to manipulate life into granting you all of your desires?

Do you become angry at objects for not doing what you expect them to do?

Do you start feeling sorry for yourself when you don't get what you want?

We're all guilty of these behaviors. But we can still give ourselves the gift of a firm footing in reality. That's the beauty of yoga: It builds strength from the ground up.

The balancing series is a perfect example. Poses like eagle, standing head to knee, standing bow, and balancing stick wake up the soles of the feet in a powerful and restorative way, teaching us to equalize our weight between the base of the big toe and baby toe and the heel. It's harder than it sounds. If too much weight is on the outside of the foot or in the heel, you slowly tip over. But once you learn to have a firm footing in reality, breathing and emptying your mind of expectation, you can live at peace.

 Are you living your life in the Now?

May 18

We're all okay.

Charles, one of the yoga instructors at the studio in my hometown, has a saying that he repeats in almost every class: *Tell yourself that you're okay by taking a breath.*

What I love about this command is how it gives us a chance to practice acceptance. Not through our words, but through our verbs. The simple act of breathing creates a full-body Yes. That's a skill that benefits every area of our lives.

Anytime we're feeling disconnected and unforgiving about ourselves, we take a breath. We stop trying to deny reality and acknowledge it instead. We remind ourselves that we're okay. And we gently carry on with our lives. Proving that when we lead with acceptance, there are no wrong moves.

 How can breathing help you practice acceptance?

May 19

Find something new every time.

Jazz musician John Coltrane's band was famous for playing the same songs in the second set as they played in the first one, just to see if they could find something they didn't find earlier in the evening. Of course, they always did. They never stepped in the same musical river twice. That's the beauty of jazz. If you do it right, redundancy becomes a mathematical impossibility. What's interesting is, the same rule can apply to our yoga practice. When we impose a baseline of curiosity and discovery and growth, practicing the discipline of seeing things with wide-open wonder, we make it easy find something new every time we're in the studio. It's all about surprise.

Neuroscientists have actually conducted mountains of research on this very issue, proving that the human brain hates boredom and loves surprises. In fact, regardless of whether or not people say they like surprises, typically life's unexpected pleasures are more rewarding than expected ones.

That's all surprise is. It's the emotion we feel when we encounter the unexpected. And if we commit to doing yoga and seeking what is fresh, spontaneous, and interesting in the same place we looked for it yesterday, nothing can strip us of myriad opportunities for wonder. Every new posture becomes an opportunity to grow closer to ourselves; to learn to understand our evolving needs as the years go by. And that's a really courageous form of growth.

 How many of your postures have enough uncertainty to make life sizzle and renew your sense of wonder?

May 20

Put your imagination to work.

Kurt Vonnegut once said that the triumph of anything is a matter of organization. I agree. But I also think that the failure of anything is a matter of imagination. It's our lack of creativity that hinders success. And unless we began taking charge of how we use our brains, we'll never achieve it.

When I'm doing yoga, I have a tendency to put the pedal to the metal inside my head. Every thought and idea, plan and problem comes thrashing to the surface at once. Most yoga experts would tell me to focus on the breath, stay in the present, and let my thoughts come and go like passing clouds in the sky.

As an experiment, I recently tried the reverse approach. Instead of attempting to force calm into my mind, I started wondering to myself, *How can I channel my thoughts into something more meaningful?* I started running creative visualizations. During class, I would use my imagination to build a story in my head. A mental movie with pictures and sounds and smells and other sensations associated with reaching a particular goal. And I would hold that fantasy until class was over.

The experience was blissful. As a result of the visualization, I was able to drown out the chatter of my mind. By tuning into the exciting movie I'd created for myself, I experienced a completely different kind of relaxation. It was a powerful example of how common wisdom isn't always exactly what we need. Do yourself the favor of finding what works best for you.

 To what extent could you let you brain race, but still be in control of it?

May 21

Let go of judgment.

Yoga changed my body and mind, but more importantly, it changed my relationship *with* my body and mind. That's the practice. In those little moments when we feel afraid and insecure and limited, we refuse to allow judgment to add fuel to the fire of our emotions. Because that only damages the relationship with ourselves further. Judging ourselves for having a problem can actually be worse than the problem itself.

Students make mistakes in postures every class. When it happens, the temptation is to berate our bodies for not doing things right in the name of high standards, because we haven't lived up to our own demands on ourselves. *Listen leg, we had a deal. I know you can rotate ninety degrees. You did it yesterday. What's your problem?*

Instead of turning on the man in the mirror in harsh judgment, let the breath take over and the muscles relax. Practice softening to the pain rather than tensing up around it. That allows us to make progress in our journey to freedom. As the recovery mantra goes, we attempt to live our lives in this manner, and we attempt to have compassion for ourselves when we don't.

That's the beauty of facing reality and transforming our relationship to it. Even if there is always a judgmental axe ready to fall, we can sidestep it once we surrender to yoga.

 What practice helps remind you that forgiveness is not something you will ever be done with?

May 22

Choose to step forward and not back.

Tell me if this sounds familiar: You're working on a train wreck of a project or managing the customer from hell. Maybe you're giving a presentation to an audience of crickets. Whatever the scenario, there's nothing you can do about it. There's no escape from your responsibilities. A cold finger of dread hooks around your heart, panic soaks your skin, and waves of anxiety start traveling up and down your spine.

It's the worst—you feel completely trapped. Paralyzed under the weight of helplessness, you think to yourself, *I just want to run away and hide from the world.* Your experience isn't even painful. Pain left town a while ago. In this space, what you're left with is a quieter, more insidious feeling. Pain's third cousin. Numbness. The anti-feeling. How can you cope?

It reminds me of a mantra we repeat at my yoga studio during some of the longer and more challenging postures: *The only way out is through.* The only option is to keep going. Our acceptance of the situation doesn't mean we approve of it, or that we like it, or that we don't want it to change. It simply means that we stop trying to deny reality and acknowledge what *is* instead. Then, we put our helplessness behind us. We go straight through the difficult moment without yielding to the urge to escape. And we go finish this thing we started, to the best of our abilities. Yes, situations can be challenging. But like the sequences, they all eventually end.

 How are you shrinking back from the path?

May 23

Find another way of moving forward.

When difficult emotions come pouring in, we're told that we have three options to cope: *fight, flight,* or *freeze.* Fighting might mean crying, punching, grinding our teeth, or arguing. Flight might mean mentally or physically running away. Freezing could be holding our breath or, my childhood preference, playing dead.

These are the three most well-documented responses to adversity, but there's a fourth option people rarely talk about: *friend.* My yoga instructor taught me this many years ago. I was going through a deeply anxious period, searching for postures to eliminate my stress, when she asked this question: *How good are you at loving your stress?* That opened my eyes to a new way of approaching anxiety. It taught me to make space for my fears. To respect them. Even start a dialogue with them during yoga class:

Well hello there fear, nice to see you again. Thank you for trying to help me today. I think I may have found another way of moving forward, and I appreciate what you're trying to do for me. Thanks for your efforts. See you next time.

It really works. Friending my emotions has been the single best strategy for diffusing stress in any situation.

When fight, flight, or freeze responses offer themselves up, try friending: Accept your difficult emotions as a part of you, give them a hug, and thank them for sharing. But then move on and get back to camel posture.

 What kind of relationship do you have with your own emotions?

May 24

Check your 'tude.

When you're in school, you don't take boring classes because the knowledge will serve you later in life, you take boring classes to master the habit of doing things you don't want to do. Because that's ninety percent of life. Doing things we don't love or even like, but trusting that we're better because of it.

Sometimes yoga can feel that way, especially in the beginning. On certain days, you're just not in the mood. There's nothing you want to do less than get into a hot room with a bunch of sweaty strangers and contort your body for ninety minutes. It's a crucial moment in the practice to decide that how we intend to live our life is more important to us than some transitory mood.

That's something my writing practice taught me many years before yoga was even part of my life. Strive to work in a productive, undramatic, regular way, with few creative tantrums and excuses about not being inspired or in the mood, and you will always get your pages done. Sticking to any habit or practice has nothing to do with desire, and everything to do with creating a desired effect. We don't have to love the thing itself, only its consequences.

 Is your practice a slave to the tyranny of moods?

May 25

✧

Take the leap into trust.

One of the great relationship breakthroughs is accepting that it's okay for other people to be angry and disappointed with us. On *their* end, we trust that they have the ability to cope with a wide array of feelings. We trust that they're not going to abandon us just because we said something that upset them. We trust the communication process and believe that a disagreement doesn't impact our connection.

On *our* end, we trust that it's not our job to prevent people from experiencing discomfort. We trust that whatever we did doesn't make us a bad person. We trust that we're good enough and that we don't have to spend our life proving ourselves.

A helpful mantra that my friend used to suggest is, *I'm doing this as an expression of my trust.* You can write it down, recite it inside your head, proclaim it to the universe, or verbally communicate it to another person. Whichever form the mantra takes, what matters is that you bring intention and conscious awareness to the process.

When I first bent backwards and extended my arms in an inverted posture, I not only had to trust that my ankles would be there waiting for my hands to grab, but also that my teacher was keeping an eye on my alignment and, if need be, would correct my posture. It took me eighteen months to build up the courage to try that posture. But thirty seconds into the pose, I knew it was worthwhile. Ever since that day, I've become much more likely to do things as an expression of my trust.

 What might assist you in building trust with yourself, with others, and with the universe?

May 26

Define what relaxation is for you.

Relaxing doesn't necessarily mean taking a long nap. It simply means doing things that calm and soothe your mind, body, and soul. In fact, the word *relax* simply means to loosen, become less formal, and decrease tension. The goal, then, is to engage in relaxation activities that are uniquely appealing to us. Whatever it takes to reach a state where we feel unburdened by this life's troubles. Relaxation is a native plant that grows in your own backyard.

The accountant who spends all day staring at numbers on a spreadsheet might relax by doing yoga. On the other hand, the novelist who works in a peaceful home office and lives inside his own head might relax by chopping wood in a field behind his house.

Where can *you* go that helps you relax best? How will you activate a unique tension-releasing experience that's inaccessible to you anywhere else? The answer won't save your life, but it will make it happier.

 Are you honoring your need for relaxation?

May 27

~∞~

Hone your observational skills.

Journaling is a process that helps us observe our own growth. Anytime we give ourselves permission to spew out every single thought that's running through our mind, from dreams to worries to fears to annoyances to ideas, we get to know ourselves better.

My day always starts with this ritual writing. It keeps me grounded, gives me a private place to ventilate, and clears away the crusty energies that have accumulated from the last twenty-four hours. Since our brains never turn off, even during exercise, maybe people need a way to document and release the many thoughts that come into their awareness during class. Let yoga be one piece of a larger project of self-attunement.

 Can you start a daily journaling practice on top of your yoga practice?

May 28

If you're the only person clapping, it's time to rethink what you're doing.

At our yoga studio, we're not interested in the sound of one hand clapping. We prefer the sound of one class clapping. That's why we give a round of applause at the end of each class. Because there's always somebody in need of encouragement.

The brand-new teacher. The first-time yogi. The injured yet determined student. The pregnant and about-to-pop mother. The former student who just came back after taking a year off. The veteran practitioner who just finished a sixty-day challenge. Or, my personal favorite, a round of applause for the seven people who managed to trudge through two feet of snow and arrive on time for the early-morning class.

That's the kind of affirmation and encouragement that brings students back, day after day. For us, applause helps create the vocabulary by which our community communicates.

 Are you practicing in an atmosphere of encouragement?

May 29

○○○

Befriend your lungs.

The concept of having a relationship with your own breath is an unexpected one. Because breathing is a natural biological function. Unless you're hyperventilating or hiking up a mountain, it's not something you typically think about. Breathing just happens.

But that's the beauty of practicing yoga. It doesn't teach you how to breathe, since all living creatures instinctively know how to do that. What it *does* do is help you understand, nurture, and transform your relationship with your breath. A very different thing.

In fact, many yoga gurus, teachers, and advocates joke that most people literally don't know how to breathe. But that's not true. Everybody knows how to breathe. Most people are just in abusive relationships with their breath. The real question to ask yourself is, if your breath were your spouse, would the two of you need counseling? If so, perhaps it's time to retrain your lungs.

 What are the benefits of retraining your breath?

May 30

Impose your own order on chaos.

How do you delete the drama that sometimes interferes with life? Often, we tap into an indispensable stabilizing element to cope. Something to anchor you when the world tries to knock the music out of you. Something to help you soar above the turmoil that surrounds you.

As a yoga student, my resource is my breath. Fast heart, slow lungs. Breathing reminds me that the more that chaos erupts around me, the deeper I need to breathe through my diaphragm.

That's how I cope calmly with inconveniences and how I avoid becoming wrapped up in passing "emergencies." By using my breath to remind myself that there *are* no emergencies. The tricky part is, human hardwiring predisposes us to react to our circumstances, which is a conditioned reflex. We have to teach ourselves to *respond* instead, which is a conscious choice.

 What small victories over circumstances does yoga afford you?

May 31

Get in touch with the source of your power.

A saying we see around the yoga community quite a bit, usually embroidered on shirts, canteens, towels, hats, mats, and the like, is *Breath is power*.

For anyone who's spent more than a few dozen hours on the mat, that statement has significant meaning. Because if there's one thing yoga teaches us, it's that there is always a way to maintain our power in a situation. All we have to do is breathe.

I remember the first time I underwent a cavity filling as a yoga student. Thanks to my new training in diaphragmatic breathing, the procedure wasn't nearly as painful or anxiety-inducing as in years past. Because now I had a healthy relationship with my breath. I knew how to maintain my power in the situation. Novocaine didn't stand a chance against me. My dentist even complimented me on my relaxed, steady, and meditative breathing during the process! Yoga really does have benefits outside of class.

 What practice keeps you in touch with the source of your power?

June 1

Relish the moment.

There's a mantra from a yoga teacher friend of mine that goes like this: *Take profit from this time.* Even if you only have a few seconds between postures or a few minutes after class, there is still value to be gained in each moment of your practice. This is a key feature that drew me into yoga immediately. The opportunity to never waste an opportunity.

When doing the poses, you can't help but learn the art of efficiency. It doesn't mean you're a robot; rather, that you make meaningful use of everything you are and everything you have. In a modern world where people worship at the altar of productivity, it's comforting to be encouraged to take five seconds to inhale, two seconds to pause, and then five seconds to exhale.

 What's your way of benefiting from every experience?

June 2

Integrate mindfulness into the chaos.

If we want to shift the paradigm of how we care for ourselves, the initial work starts inside of our heads. Sometimes it can feel like a sea of voices clamoring for a hearing. Like a psychic torture machine created just to make us miserable. And we know that if we don't create a wise relationship to it, it will continue to push us around.

Karen Reed, a teacher at our studio, has a great saying: *The brain is a bad neighborhood. Stay out of it.* That's good advice whether you practice yoga or not. The good news is, mindfulness is always available to us as a tool to settle the mind. It's effective, free, healthy, and simple. Mindfulness is certainly a smarter strategy than eating an entire box of oatmeal cookies to medicate our unwanted reality.

It's all about giving ourselves more options about how to act when we feel our triggers. My therapist called this *nipping anxiety in the bud*. He taught me not to worry about doing anything with the thoughts that flooded my mind, but rather, to just try to stay with them.

He also taught me that anytime we get caught in a tortuous sequence of thoughts with no apparent way out, the first step is to calmly say to ourselves, *Oh, would you look at that, there appears to be some anxiety here, interesting.* By catching our restless thoughts and separating ourselves from indulging in them, we find a peaceful route out of that bad neighborhood and float into the wide-open space of calm.

Have you developed the ability to calm the mind on demand?

June 3

Disengage from your neuroses.

The word *neurosis* derives from the Greek word for "nerves." Clinically, it's defined as a relatively mild mental illness involving irrational stress, anxiety, obsessive behavior. But it's the existential point of view posited by theologian Paul Tillich that resonates with me most: neuroses are nothing more than our anxious attempts to control life. After all, the human brain is an anticipation machine. For me, it kicks into high gear during yoga class. Whatever happens is just a trigger for me to think, *Wait, how dare my body not execute this posture perfectly?* But before shaking our hands at the sky, we might consider the wisdom of history's great thinkers.

Buckminster Fuller said that nature does not depend on us because we are not the only experiment.

Byron Katie said that the rose blooms without our approval and dies without our consent.

Fyodor Dostoyevsky said that nature doesn't ask our advice, and she isn't interested in our preferences or whether or not we approve of her laws, and so, we must accept nature as she is with all the consequences that this implies.

Knowing that the world operates on laws beyond our control, we need more skills for coping with what we cannot change. Psychologist Martin Seligman's research on human flourishing suggests that the knowledge of the difference between what we can change and what we must accept in ourselves is the beginning of real change.

 Are you ready to accept the world as it is?

June 4

Internalize a set of healthy responses and behaviors.

Hot yoga is about sweating, but it's also about surprise. Doing the postures trains our bodies to move in ways that once seemed impossible or uncomfortable. I'll never forget my first class. A guy who bent his legs like a medieval contortionist. A girl whose body looked like a waterslide. In front of me was the teacher, who I'm pretty sure was levitating. I thought there was no way I could do anything like that.

Yet one or five or ten years into the practice, few things feel unattainable. Because the progress never stops. You're always making micro-improvements. And you don't even realize it until, one random night, you're balancing your entire body weight on your palms for thirty seconds straight without even blinking. Plus, after enough time of establishing a continuous rhythm in the studio, yoga's structure of faithfully returning to challenging postures is easily applicable in other situations off the mat.

You become calm in moments that used to leave you feeling out of place and inferior. You understand how to handle conflict that once bewildered you. You find inner resources that you didn't know you had. You stand up for yourself where you're usually weak. You learn to turn inward where you formerly needed external validation. And you take bold action in situations where fear once paralyzed you.

As your yoga practice continues, trust that your body is internalizing its lessons. Know that you are carrying it inside of you as a tool for sustaining and connecting with other parts of your life. You might surprise yourself.

 What have you achieved that you used to believe was impossible?

June 5

Extend your yoga beyond class hours.

Karmasoft is an online management software program developed by the owner of my yoga studio. Roody Senecal created it because he wanted a system that connected fitness teachers with their students at the speed of conversation. My favorite feature of the program is the after-class emails. By the time we get home from practice, there's a message waiting in our inbox from the instructor:

> *Monday rock stars, great work tonight! Here's to moving forward this week with the same focus, poise, and compassion each one of you demonstrated on your mats.*

More and more studios are starting to communicate with their communities in this way. I practice yoga around the world and have seen a variety of useful tools and technologies like this one. It does my heart good, because studios are finally understanding that the yoga starts well before class begins, and continues well after class ends.

 How are you giving others the feelings of belonging that they have been seeking for so long?

June 6

Invite your inner strength to move through you.

The men in my family are prone to *vasovagal reaction*, which is a sudden drop in heart rate and blood pressure, often in reaction to a stressful trigger like blood, needles, graphic stories, and occasionally zombie movies. It's an awful feeling. Dizziness, nausea, and even fainting are just a few of the delightful symptoms. It's been a struggle of mine since adolescence.

What's fascinating is that yoga has helped me better handle this reaction. The practice has trained me to use my breath to get to a place of safety on a moment's notice. As my instructors say, wherever it hurts, send your breath there.

Nowadays, whether I'm giving blood, having painful dental work done, listening to a gross story, or sitting in the hospital to visit a sick loved one, simply being able to breathe helps me gain control over that reaction. A deep breath invites inner strength to move through me. And on a good day, it feels like I can handle anything. Take that, genetics.

 What helps you get to a place of safety on a moment's notice?

June 7

Leave your comfort zone.

It's fascinating to try out new yoga studios while traveling. There's something magical about practicing in a new city with new surroundings and new teachers. It snaps you out of your normal routines and enables you to see yourself in a new light, quite literally.

It certainly requires more time and money investment than working out in the hotel fitness center, but the people you meet, the lessons you learn, and the new terrain you explore is always meaningful. Isn't that better than the hotel fitness center? Even if you get lost on the way there and show up two minutes before class begins.

 What's your favorite way to snap out of your own routines?

June 8

It doesn't always feel better, but it always gets better.

After taking a few thousand yoga classes in the past ten years, there isn't an emotion that hasn't run through my mind before, during, or after my practice.

Rage. Sadness. Apathy. Depression. Soreness. Joy. Dehydration. Anger. Empowerment. Confusion. Numbness. Arousal. Tingling. Nausea. Dizziness. Connection. Invincibility.

Yoga makes you feel all the feels, whether you want to or not. And that's a good thing. Especially for those of us emotional neophytes who are trying out the full range of our feelings for the first time. That's the kooky thing about the head and the heart. They don't always agree with each other. And so, just because we feel something in our bodies, that doesn't mean that's who we are. And just because we're not thrilled with the emotions that arise during class, that doesn't mean we're not making progress.

It all comes down to trust. Both in ourselves and in the process. Knowing that if we keep showing up and doing the work, it will be worthwhile in the end. No matter what crazy story our bodies have to tell.

 What first gave you the courage to feel all of your feelings?

June 9

Listen for the voice of change.

There's an old Zen koan that goes something like this: *To change the course of a stream, put a pebble near its source, rather than a boulder downstream.* It's an elegant reminder that we don't have to make change any more difficult and complicated than it already is. It's simply a matter of energy and intention. It all depends on how willing we are to let go and open our hearts.

Hot yoga opened my heart in every sense of the term. Postures like camel, standing bow, and cobra have done wonders for me. They're chest openers, stretching the entire front of the body and releasing tension in the torso and neck. With the studio kept at a breezy one hundred degrees, there's no shortage of heart opening during each class. This flexibility also translates to the rest of my life. After a decade of practicing yoga, I find hearing the voice of change isn't as hard as it used to be thanks to a more open heart and flexible body.

I now search for the paths that lead to change, meeting each challenge as an opportunity to explore my strengths. It turns out that most change is gentle and undramatic, and that seeing how I am changing is exciting and encouraging, even when it's slow. Change is still scary, but with yoga as the pebble at the source of the stream, it's much easier to control the flow of the water and direct the energy in a positive direction.

 What intention might inspire you to become more trusting of change?

June 10

It's human to fall out, it's yoga to get back in.

Any new way of living requires much practice, but it also requires an equal measure of perseverance. Thankfully, that's what yoga teaches. We learn to be gentle with ourselves, patient in our efforts, and forgiving of our failures. And even when we can't touch our toes or lift our legs or even face our bodies in the mirror, we keep listening to the rhythm of our spirit.

Balancing in standing head-to-knee pose comes to mind. Bikram calls this pose a *ten-year posture*. That's how much perseverance it requires. One day the knee fully locks out and your elbows swing wildly down. The next day your standing leg wobbles and shifts your body weight onto your outer foot until you plié off your mat like a drunken ballerina.

And that's okay. It's human to fall out of posture, it's yoga to jump back in.

 How can you contribute to your reserve of patience?

June 11

Your body is just where you live right now.

Buddhist teacher Noah Levine's inspiring manifesto about mindfulness and awakening, *The Heart of the Revolution,* makes a brilliant observation that the body is not who we are, it is just what we are currently experiencing. That quotation should be framed and hung on the wall of every yoga studio on the planet.

Because each time we do our practice, our bodies are different from the day before. They might be sore, tired, bloated, bruised, flexible, dehydrated, hungover, stressed out, or straight-up injured. But that's not who we are. It's just the packaging. Sanskrit has a beautiful phrase for this, *aham sakish,* which translates to *I am the eternal witness.*

Meaning, there is the innermost self that lives on, but everything else, including our thoughts and cells of our body, is transitory. When we stare at our bodies in the mirror and start berating ourselves for being imperfect we must remember: Your body is not who you are, it's just where you live right now. Think of it like the weather. If you don't like it, just wait an hour.

 Are you respecting your body, or fighting it?

June 12

Rise into union.

The word *yoga* literally translates to mean "union." The integration of the mind, body, and spirit. Throughout your practice, there are many examples of this union. For example, as long as we are in conflict with our body, we cannot find peace of mind. But when we learn to listen to what our muscles and joints are telling us, when we accept our physical limitations, our anxiety magically begins to dissipate and our mind becomes clearer. That's union.

Here's another example: During the balancing postures, we keep our eyeballs still and focus on a single point, either in the mirror, on the ceiling, or along the carpet. This quiets our mind, keeps the body fixed, and deepens our connection of spirit. That's union. It's not so much about balance as it is about integration. Mind, body, and spirit, working together as one.

 What are the ways your practice is integrated?

June 13

Don't be ashamed to feel good.

It was summer, at rush hour, in a sold-out class with forty sweaty strangers working their minds, bodies, and spirits into amazing condition. When we finished the last posture and keeled over into final savasana, our teacher said something that had a profound impact on me. Robin reminded us: *It's not shameful to feel this good.*

In that moment, some tightly wrapped coil of stress let go inside of us. The room felt palpably different. All of a sudden, all of our guilt and shame floated out of our bodies as we allowed ourselves to soak up the feelings of joy and invigoration that we rightly deserved.

 Are you allowing life to flow abundantly through you?

June 14

Actions are only dangerous when done dangerously.

I once read an interview with a world-famous mountain climber, Conrad Anker. The guy had just finished scaling seven of the world's largest peaks in one year's time, and the journalist asked him the one question we sane people were wondering:

Is mountain climbing dangerous? His answer made me smile: "It's only dangerous if you do it dangerously." Says the man who lost three fingers and his best friend to frostbite.

And yet, there's still wisdom in his response. Because yoga, like any activity or sport, is also only dangerous when done dangerously. If you come to class hungover, sick with the flu, or just trying to win a bet that you can last longer than your roommate, it's a recipe for disaster. You may not get frostbite, but you'd still be better off taking a step back.

 How might you be making the yoga air heavy with the weight of dangerous possibilities?

June 15

Get hot in the studio, not in your temper.

Here's my favorite cheesy saying from the twelve-step recovery movement: Time is an acronym for *This I must earn.* When it comes to yoga, this idea couldn't be more applicable. Because yoga is a highly patient practice. You can't win the whole world on the first day. Some poses take years to even try, much less master. All you can do is make progress, inch by inch, posture by posture, trusting that each movement is gradually moving your mind and body toward some kind of enlightenment.

Fortunately, the patience you display on the yoga mat also makes a powerful statement that you are not judging others or yourself too harshly. I remember a teacher once telling us during an insanely humid summer class: *Listen guys, this yoga is so hot, you won't have time to lose your cool.*

We weren't sure if that was a riddle, a Zen koan, or another meaningless platitude, but either way, the teacher's words made everyone in the class smile. It felt like she had created a spaciousness in the room by acknowledging everybody's frustration. In a world where most people's patience is hanging at the other end of a very thin thread, that's not an insignificant accomplishment.

 When was the last time your impatience got the best of you?

June 16

Yoga practice, not yoga perfect.

It's yoga practice, not yoga perfect. That's the mantra that reminds us we're human and flawed and doing the best we can. On and off the mat. We're all dented cans, faulty vessels aspiring to a new wholeness.

Each time we fall out of posture, slip on the mat, knock over our water bottle, or show up to class late, we must forgive ourselves and let it go. We remember that whatever mistake we just made, odds are, the other twenty students doing yoga in the same room have done the same thing, multiple times over.

Perfect is for amateurs. Perfect is the burden that keeps you from true growth. Focus on practicing. Practice is the most reliable vehicle for change. Practice is what allows you to float nimbly through yoga from one day to the next.

 What do you need to trade in your perfectionism for?

June 17

Jump off the trauma train.

Big or small, mental and emotional scars from past distressing experiences are something we all have. From that point forward, we are especially attuned to reminders of our suffering. Any stimuli can become a trigger. It might be loud noises for one person, airplane turbulence for another, or an unreachable partner for a third.

At the height of my workaholic years, I was driven by the fear that if I didn't work sixteen hours a day and travel nonstop, I would lose my job and become a failure and have to go crawling back to my parents' basement as a broke, lonely, and pathetic loser.

It was a textbook workaholic mindset. It even sent me to the hospital several times for stress-related injuries, including a collapsed lung. To heal, I started yoga and did whatever else it took. But the thing about trauma is, the body has a long memory. Things like working and traveling and even certain people are still associated with pain and stress for me. Sometimes, we have to specifically work to get comfortable again. As much as our brain loves to jump at reminders of a scary event, the threat is gone now. Yoga helps me do that by reminding me to breathe through my fear.

 How can you set your brain free from fear?

June 18

Keep the door open to progress.

It's not about our performance of the posture, but our commitment to progress. That's the only thing worth measuring. Are we growing? Are we deepening? Are we different people than we were when we first started the practice?

Martín Prechtel said it best in his book about apprenticing as a shaman, *The Unlikely Peace at Cuchumaquic*: "There is no finish line, no heaven-like last act, no glorious arrival. There is only the glorious continuation."

Try not to put too much pressure on yourself to be the greatest, be the best, or be perfect. Focus on the small wins that enable you to continue the journey a little bit each day.

 Do you have a compulsive obsession with perfection, or a remarkable devotion to progress?

June 19

Form a positive addiction.

I'm a big believer in the power of positive addiction. Recently a newcomer at my yoga studio asked if practicing daily would have a negative psychological impact. I told her it was the opposite. Getting yourself hooked on healthy, meaningful routines is always a wise investment. These types of positive addictions create extremely optimal conditions for us to flourish. Unlike other addictions, they rarely get you arrested or divorced.

It might be hot yoga, or going for a run, or making a cup of tea each evening, or taking soothing baths. The trick is to make your body crave the ritual. After a while, it actually becomes easier to stick with the practice than to skip it. That's the secret to positive addiction. Building habit, building discipline, and getting to the point where you feel worse when you don't do something. Not a bad corner to paint yourself into.

 What are you positively addicted to?

June 20

Keep your mind on your mat.

The hardest advice to take is to keep our minds on our mats. We'd much rather meddle in other people's business.

Look at that guy next to the mirror. Why does he keep talking to himself?

That lady sitting down by the back door: Is she going to pass out?

What about the instructor? How about opening a window in this sauna of a studio?

Does the dude in front of me know that there's a giant hole in the seat of his pants? I think he just smiled at me.

Can somebody please tell the guy in the front row to pull up his shorts, for God's sake?

None of these ruminations makes our practice any better. Only more distracted. If we truly want to get the most out of our yoga, it's best to keep our eyes on our own mat. No matter how annoying, bizarre, fascinating, or beautiful the people around us are. The only thing that matters is the person staring back at us in the mirror.

 What distractions will you avoid today?

June 21

Do yoga long enough, and watch your life change.

How long do you have to practice yoga before seeing meaningful benefits? This is at the top of every frequently asked questions list on yoga websites.

The fortune cookie answer is: Practice is the most reliable vehicle for change.

The inspiring answer is: Even at your fairly immature level of practice, you will already feel yoga's potency.

The empowering answer is: You will gain some benefit from the very first breath.

The Zen answer is: You will start to see benefits when you stop looking for them.

The football coach answer is: The harder you work, the faster you'll grow.

The inclusive answer is: Everybody and every body is different, so there's really no way to tell.

The frustrating answer is: Probably longer than you expect.

The peaceful answer is: Forget about how long it will take and just enjoy the journey.

The scriptural answer is: Yoga is the journey of the self, through the self, to the self.

The incrementalist answer is: There will be small but perceptible increases, until one day you're suddenly able to bend your head and kiss the curve of your own neck.

Confused? Don't be. The only answer that counts is the one you provide yourself.

 How does your perspective on the benefits of yoga inform your answers?

June 22

Tune into the world around you.

Silent yoga classes challenge students to be their own teachers. In the absence of the instructor's dialogue to cue, guide, and correct postures, the practice becomes blissfully quiet and, more importantly, completely autonomous. Language processing uses up a lot of your brain's bandwidth. In a silent class, there's nothing to listen to except your body. Your inner voice. Your intuitive faculties.

Yoga instructors often report that during silent classes, very few students sit out. Or leave the room. Or look around to compare themselves to others. Or pace around their mats in a drama-filled tantrum. They're too focused and present with their own practice. What's more, without teacher commands, students are forced to align their bodies to the communal energy of the room. Intuiting entrances and exits to postures based on the shared movements around them and becoming more connected to their environment. Like a school of fish that moves collectively, communicating via something other than spoken language.

I've participated in dozens of silent classes in studios around the world, and they never fail to take my practice to new heights. They challenge me to reduce my dependence on an external locus of control, which makes me feel empowered and efficacious. And they flood my brain with new ideas for my business that I never would have created if I were busy listening to the teacher. Know when to use your voice, but more importantly, know when to use your silence.

 Are you willing to welcome every layer of silence?

June 23

Launch the anxiety reduction subroutine.

Yoga is one of many strategies that I employ to manage my anxiety in a healthy way. It works in part because practicing is an aerobic activity that boosts my brain's dopamine levels and provides endorphins, but also because my studio is a supportive community of compassionate people.

We all struggle and thrive, fail and persevere on the mat together, even if we don't know each other's names, even if we don't know each other's lives outside the hot room. Anytime I find myself shrouded in a cloud of melancholy, it's simply a matter of launching the anxiety reduction subroutine by returning to my yoga community. Works every time.

 How does yoga help you manage anxiety?

June 24

Awareness, not avoidance.

When things hurt, instead of trying to camouflage your agony, my yoga instructor would tell you to try sending your breath to the pain. Before taking any other action, fill your lungs deeply and send your breath to where it stings.

To thread your breath through every action helps maintain a sense of inner control in the midst of outer chaos. It cultivates a state of mind that fosters equanimity and forbearance. That in turn helps you find the inner fortitude to navigate even the most devastating storms.

 How do you use your breath to soothe yourself?

June 25

Change your response to the struggles of life.

In many ways, addiction and yoga are polar opposites. One is leaving the moment; the other is checking in with it. One is trying to change or control our feelings and thoughts and emotions; the other is learning to accept them. One is doing whatever it takes to get anywhere but where we are; the other is trying to get the most out of what's in our mind, body, and spirit right now.

One is motivated by the fear of pain; the other deepens our awareness and tolerance of it. One is a hell we get trapped in; the other is a haven that's always there for us to return to. One is a tempting but ineffective way to handle recurrent crises of meaning; the other is a healthy vehicle for connecting with self and others.

The list goes on, and that's a good thing. Because in the last ten years, yoga has been a godsend in helping me heal my wounds, compulsions, and dependencies. Yours may look different from mine, but we all lean too much on a bad habit for comfort in times of need, whether it's binge-watching TV, surfing the internet for hours, eating food that doesn't make us feel good, throwing ourselves into work, or any other avoidance tactic. Replace any of our addictive behaviors with yoga and we find ourselves taking steps away from compulsive behavior and into mindful practice.

 What helps you choose healthier ways of de-stressing?

June 26

Pursue intimacy.

In the handbook of addictive disorders used by clinicians, expert psychologists explain that intimacy is incompatible with workaholism, and that a workaholic is anyone who uses busyness to avoid getting in touch with personal feelings and stay clear of intimacy. That was me in spades. Thinking back to my entrepreneurial twenties, when fourteen-hour days were the norm, my tendency was to stubbornly do everything myself, and to romanticize my professional exertions as a form of heroism.

It was awesome for my business, but awful for my relationships. Working all the time gave me a perfect excuse to not have time for other people. Good people. Loving people. People who were trying to get close enough that they might actually see what I was trying to hide. Fortunately, a mentor helped me realize the importance of beginning a journey of reconnecting to the world.

A critical part of that process was joining my local yoga community. Turns out, taking cues from the teacher, working together with your fellow yogis, and performing the postures in unison with the class are all brilliant tools for learning the value of shared effort and cooperative spirit. Yoga not only gave me a brief respite from work, it also created much-needed moments of connection and belonging with others. If you're struggling with an addiction or a compulsion that keeps you clear of intimacy, try getting on the mat. It's a surprisingly powerful first step.

 How do you intentionally create experiences that force you to collaborate with other people?

June 27

Strive for balance.

Striking the balance between relaxation and exertion on the mat equips you to drop deeper into the posture. Strain too hard, and you may overshoot the mark. Don't reach far enough, and you can't attain the shape. It's easy to remind yourself not to do the latter, but most of us still err when it comes to overextending ourselves.

But what if you're starting a business? Or creating an art piece? Or beginning a new relationship? The same principle applies. Relax and exert simultaneously. Learn to ask yourself: *What unused, underleveraged component of this process can I engage while waiting for the paint to dry elsewhere?*

Sometimes, straining toward your fullest extension isn't as effective as relaxing into it.

 Can you be impatient and patient at the same time?

June 28

Learn to see things dispassionately.

Vital to yoga is the ability to breathe with a slow, relaxed pace. Many newcomers and first-timers miss the mark on this practice, but more experienced yogis can lose sight of it as well. As soon as their muscles start to hurt, or the sweat rolls down their skin, enter the cardiovascular drama. They'll default to shallow, rapid, and dramatic breathing through their chest rather than from their center. Though they may think it will help them move through the posture, it only makes it worse.

What you learn in yoga is that the faster your heart beats, the slower your lungs need to fill. The more that chaos erupts around you, the deeper you need to breathe through your diaphragm. It's a metaphor for life. Reacting dramatically to internal and external turmoil is universal but unhelpful. You need to practice breathing through it instead. Only when you put your emotions and racing breath aside can you evaluate your situation objectively. Only then can you respond, not react, from a space of peace.

 Through what lens do you view your situations?

June 29

Make sure you are in touch with what you really need.

When you're wired for hard work, the hardest thing to do is nothing. The opposite of ambition. The antithesis of labor. Idleness. *Blech*. But just like in the yoga room, where the posture you *hate* the most is the posture you *need* the most, doing nothing is often the right move. Think of it this way: Sabbatical comes from the word *sabbath*, meaning "day of rest." The practice dates back to ancient agriculture and Mosaic law, which decreed that every seventh year a farmer's land was to remain untilled while debtors and slaves were to be released. Maybe that's what you need. To leave the land alone. To emancipate yourself as a slave to achievement.

So a few summers ago, I decided to do nothing for three straight months. *No working. No writing. No marketing. No strategizing. No nothing.* Just a lot of sleeping, a lot of walking, a lot of reading, a lot of singing, and a lot of traveling. And cookies. Oh man were there cookies.

It turns out, for someone who's theoretically happiest when he's productive and prolific, taking a sabbatical was the best thing I could have done. By the time summer was over, I was rejuvenated and equipped for the next chapter of life. What I thought I couldn't stand was exactly what I needed.

 When was the last time you took time off to recharge?

June 30

Leverage your energy.

Breathe through it is what we're told on the mat. According to yoga, every posture, difficult as it may seem, can always be navigated effectively if you just breathe through it.

Breath is always the secret—for the postures, and for the rest of our life. Channel your energy into something more productive than your racing thoughts or anxieties. Think back to everything meaningful you've created in your life. Odds are, some energy force compelled you to take action.

It's simply a matter of channeling that energy strategically. Use the breath, and the impossible suddenly seems within reach. It might be a tricky balancing posture, or it might be something you've long wanted to manifest in your personal or professional life. Once you have your breath, it's time to reach out for your goals.

 How can you use your breath to bring the impossible within reach?

July 1

Start appreciating your shortcomings.

There's no need to panic at the thought of our own weaknesses. They're worth making friends with. In fact, once we know what they are, and once we're willing to face them head on, these weaknesses can actually become strengths.

During WWII, a small number of aerial observers were specifically recruited by the United States Air Force because they were colorblind. Turns out, they were able to distinguish camouflaged military equipment. Thanks to their "disability," their eyes were never fooled. It made them an invaluable asset to the organization.

It's an interesting paradox, considering that we live in such a winning-is-everything, only-the-strong-survive culture. We overlook the value of our weaknesses, assuming they're best discounted or deleted instead of located and loved. The secret: this weakness, this vulnerability, can actually become our strongest weapon. It's simply a matter of mental framing, of changing the story we tell ourselves about our limitations.

Yogis learn to love and listen to and leverage the body they've been given. They discover which postures are easier and more enjoyable to execute, *because* of the very weaknesses they used to hide from. That often invites smiles and admiration from fellow students, proving that limitations are the doorways to our deepest value. They're always worth making friends with. The best part is, endorsing our own weakness establishes our acceptance of the imperfect humanness of others.

 How might you take what should have held you back and use it to move forward?

July 2

Listen for the word, not the tone.

Yoga is, at its core, a practice of active listening. To our bodies, to the room, to our fellow students, and to our instructor. The hard part is discerning the signal from the noise. Without such a distinction, our practice gets rooted in expectation, as opposed to awareness. And that robs us of the present moment. Robin, our studio's preacher/teacher hybrid, constantly reminds us during class: Try to listen for the word, not the tone.

If you hear the prefix *ch-*, don't come out of the posture three seconds early, anticipating the word *change*. Your instructor might be about to say chest or chin, which could have been a valuable correction for your pose. So instead of making assumptions, be patient in your transitions and wait to act on direction.

 How has yoga made you a better listener?

July 3

Breathe in tandem.

With the exception of a few dozen solo sessions in hotel rooms, saunas, and gyms, most of my yoga has been done in a group. It's just not the same when I'm alone. For me, that's a good thing. Because at a certain point in your life, you don't need more you. True growth only happens in the presence of other people. During final breathing our instructors say, listen to the sound of the breath, and know you're not alone.

It's a simple yet soothing reminder that when we do this yoga practice, we are richly supported and connected. In fact, that's the slogan for my studio, Yoga Tribe Brooklyn: Every. Body. Belongs. We're not nearly as powerful in isolation as we are together.

 What helps remind you that you're not alone?

July 4

Look for your special light.

Everyone has hard classes. Days when you start sweating before the first posture. Or your body doesn't bend the way it did last week. Or when you wolf down two bags of potato chips on the train ride to class. Or when your limbs are so tired that you can hardly move. Or when your brain starts racing about that important project and you have to fight the urge to duck out of class and check your email in the locker room.

The adorable part about these so-called hard classes is that we all think we're unique in our suffering. That nobody else understands how hard it is for us. Next time you catch yourself looking around the room to see if anybody notices just how hard it is for you, consider asking this question instead:

Is this problem really a crisis, or just another one of the ongoing issues that confronts all people? It's probably the latter. Welcome to the human race. Where even if you're not unique, at least you're not alone.

 What would it look like to put something besides your problems at the center of your life today?

July 5

Embrace the diversity of breath.

The one truth most yogis can agree on is that if you lose your breath you lose your practice. Here are a few of my favorite metaphors explaining this:

Breath is the thread that ties your practice together.

Breath is the teacher, telling you what you can do and helping to guide you.

Breath is the fuel source, the subtlest way to gain energy, a natural source of oxygen.

Breath is the bridge between your mind, body, and soul.

Breath is the language through which your mind, body, and soul communicate, building the fluency of knowing the self.

Breath is the friend, always available to you in every situation.

Breath is the metronome, allowing you to keep time and enjoy learning the postures.

Breath is the medicine, the body's most natural way to help you stay present, calm, focused, and in control.

Breath is the conversation with the world, the most immediate and intimate way of engaging with everything around you.

Ultimately, it doesn't matter what we call the breath, only that we use it.

 What metaphor best deepens your relationship with your breath?

July

July 6

Find a studio that shares your values.

Years ago I read an advertisement in the back of a yoga journal that said the following: Come do yoga in a gently heated loft space. Noncompetitive atmosphere. Fall in love with yourself. Beginners welcome.

Speaking as both a yoga student and a marketer, that's smart copywriting. The product is attractive, inclusive, and empowering. A place where every yoga class is a fresh opportunity to love ourselves a little bit more, and to judge ourselves a little bit less? Where the goal is accepting ourselves, not achieving skinny waistlines? *Yes, please.*

But yoga is about more than a studio sales package. Is where you practice living up to its promises? Make sure that your community is one you want to be part of. Even if that means occasionally switching lanes as your needs change.

 What would a yoga advertisement have to say to get you in the door?

July 7

Loving ourselves is not an indulgence.

Time after time, multiple instructors have given me the same advice about the practice of yoga: Loving ourselves is the primary lesson we are here to learn.

Yes, bending and stretching and flexing are the surface-level actions, but underneath those physical moves is a baseline of emotional development. Like those days when we're feeling fat and worthless, and we still manage to come to class and confront ourselves in the mirror and accept whatever we see. Or those days when we can't seem to do anything right at work, we feel incompetent and likely to get fired any day now, but we still show up and do the postures and honor whatever level of skill we've been given.

If we can still love ourselves in those situations, that's a victory that ripples out into the rest of our lives. As the mat goes, so goes the world. Because yoga is, at its fundamental level, another way to practice being kind to ourselves in small, concrete ways.

 What is the primary lesson yoga has taught you?

July 8

Become friends with your weaknesses.

In hatha yoga (the form most Western studios practice), we perform a series of postures in which we balance on one foot at a time. These poses are long and demanding, calling upon tremendous strength in the core and leg muscles, as well as developing our concentration and determination.

Beyond the muscle benefits, the real advantage of doing postures that require balance is that they bring us up against our limitations in an immediate way. These poses tell us where we need to grow. Years ago my therapist taught me to ask the question: How can I make friends with this feeling? For example, my core has always been pretty weak. In the balancing pose *dandayamana janushirasana* (standing head to knee), kicking my leg straight out and touching my head to my knee very rarely happens. And that's okay. The posture helps me make friends with my weakness. It reminds me to suck in my gut and keep the core engaged, and I'm grateful for that struggle. It's what helps me grow.

 How are you using weakness as a potent purifier?

July 9

Create room for the new.

Yoga is a glorious release valve. The postures allow you to release your grip on your own body, and open your hands to receive the new. Because it focuses on the *now*, you have to let go of *before*.

It's a beautiful give-and-take system. Each time you stumble, new strength is gained. Each time you fail, new knowledge is ingrained. Each time you show up and do the work, new milestones are attained. Each time you return to the mat committed to learning something new about yourself, new facets of identity are unchained.

Turn the release valve, and you might be surprised to find inner resources you didn't know you had. Let go of the limitation you've been tightly gripping, and you'll be amazed what will come into your hands.

 Are you ready to release your grip on the past and open your palms to receive the new?

July 10

Make progress, not perfection.

Bikram Choudhury constantly reminds his students that few of us ever do the poses perfectly. Instead, it's about how well you understand what you're trying to accomplish in each pose and how you try to accomplish your goal. You don't just learn the ideal pose, you learn what challenges you will face during the process, in addition to what clues will help you make rapid progress. As a student myself, I've achieved powerful results by embracing this principle in my own practice. Turns out, progress revolves around asking yourself these three questions:

How do you gauge progress?

What amount of progress is acceptable?

Can you think of a way to quantify that amount so you can constantly measure it?

That will focus you on moving forward without worrying about moving flawlessly.

 Are you trying to keep from losing ground, or trying to make progress?

July 11

Go deeper.

Yoga is recreational, but it's also relational. Between the mind, body, and soul. Between the ego and the self. Between the individual and the community. Between the conscious and subconscious. Between the old version of our being and the new model. Between the ideal dream and the grounded reality.

It all begins with the breath. It's the celestial cord that binds various entities together. Eric Maisel, my favorite meditation teacher, said it best:

> When we consciously decide to breathe more slowly and deeply, we alert our body to the fact that we want it to behave differently. We are not just changing our breathing pattern; we are making a full-body announcement that we are entering into a different relationship with our mind and body.

I used to have a yoga teacher who sounded like a broken record every time she asked students her trademark question: How's your breathing? Her repetition was no accident. She was trying to help us focus on the unseen, not just the motions.

 What kind of relationship do you have with your breath?

July 12

~⚬~

Mess with the gods, not with your knees.

Before I fell in love with yoga, running was my favorite form of exercise. It was a relaxing, joyful, and portable practice for staying healthy and sane. Then my knees and ankles started to give out. To the point where the pain of running slowly outweighed the benefits, even though the salesman at the running store told me: *There's no such thing as bad joints, only bad gear.*

It's a good closing sales pitch (even if the biology is suspect), but I went on running hiatus during the winter season anyway, and as luck would have it, yoga came into my life at around the same time. Unlike running, it actually did wonders for my sore joints. After my first class, I never looked back. It's certainly not the same thing as jogging through a forest on a hot, rainy night with nobody around but me and the stars, but ultimately, my body thanks me for it. We have to make sure we're listening to our own injuries first, before we listen to those who think they know better.

 Which of your favorite practices have you outgrown?

July 13

Create golden moments.

Anything that enables a blissful sense of expansive oneness with others, with new ideas and experiences, is a worthwhile use of our time. As those little everyday moments add up we can build a bank of resilience with them. In those moments, we need a reminder that sometimes we've been amazed and awed by our life. C. S. Lewis wrote about this phenomenon in his book *Surprised by Joy*:

> *This really was a period of ecstasy that consisted chiefly of moments when you were too happy to speak, when the gods and heroes rioted through your head until you felt that it might break you with mere richness.*

Lewis had that sensation during one of the darker times in his life, when he was away at a boarding school he disliked and took refuge in books. It's a lesson for us all that even in bleak surroundings, we can find a source of pleasure. Are you pulling your triggers for joy and committing daily acts that evoke aliveness? Are you learning to find satisfaction in the little things?

Yoga does that for me every single day. Even if I sit out half the postures. Because every life needs moments of exultation. Any small gesture or tiny embellishment that has a memorable impact on us is a sign that we're still alive. Each of us deserves to have moments so golden that they take our breath away. Each of us deserves an environment that conveys a sense of wholeness and evokes a quality of aliveness. It doesn't have to be yoga, it just has to be yours.

 Are you orienting yourself toward that which delights you?

July 14

Reject preconceptions.

When I first started practicing yoga, I would keep track of how many days in a row I made it to the studio. It made me feel strong at first. But after a while, the number started creating an expectation. I would think to myself, well, now that ten days have passed, I bet my body will start to fatigue.

Sure enough, the next day I would leap out of bed with searing calf cramps and race to the fridge to suck back coconut waters until the pain subsided. So much for feeling strong. In order to flourish, I had to stop expecting my body to hit a wall.

It reminds me of the words of Dana Torres, the oldest swimmer ever to earn a place on the U.S. Olympic Team. She said the water doesn't know how old you are. Funny what's possible when we stop making gods out of numbers and stop limiting our expectations.

 What numbers or ideas are holding back your practice?

July 15

Moving at the speed of the soul, and not any faster.

Hillary Clinton was an inspiring leader long before she ran as the first female presidential candidate nominated by a major political party. Back in the sixties, she delivered a moving commencement address at her alma mater, Wellesley College. Here's the quote that stuck out for me: *Fear is always with us, but we just don't have time for it.* It's a poignant yet practical concept that reinforces the human necessity for movement. How we must keep moving forward, even when we're scared.

Hot yoga was instrumental in teaching me this very skill. Ask anyone who's practiced before. The series of poses is so relentless, there's no room for fear. The instructor fills nearly every minute with the fluid and fast instructions for the class, and all you have time to do is follow the words, set up the postures, shift into awkward balancing positions, fall out, and then start over again.

Our fears may be with us, but we simply don't have time for them. It's like a line out of the eighties action movie *Predator*. One soldier says to his partner, *Hey man, you're shot, and you're bleeding!* To which the reply is, *I ain't got time to bleed.* The courage to reach past our fear is within us. We just need to move fast enough to distract ourselves.

 What actions might banish the fears that undermine your courage?

July 16

Embrace the intangible.

Acts of forgiveness, kindness, acceptance, and compassion can't be measured. There's no conversion rate, no return on investment, and no reliable metric to prove that our emotional efforts were a prudent use of our time. They still matter, though. Albert Einstein kept a sign in his office that displayed the following phrase: *Not everything that matters can be measured, and not everything that is measured matters.*

A perfect mantra for the hard work of training the heart. Where we trust that every act of love pays a dividend and every meditative effort brings us one step closer to joy. Even if we can't measure the progress, we shall not labor in vain.

Yoga has become my favorite venue for doing this work. Every day when I practice, my body inevitably falls out of posture. Dozens and dozens of times. But instead of rolling my eyes and shaking my head and cursing under my breath about what a clumsy doughboy I am, the braver response is to laugh it off and feel proud of my effort and hop back in to try it again.

Bikram likes to say that falling out of a posture means you are human, but getting back into the posture means you are a yogi. That's the real yoga. Acting toward ourselves with love. Reminding ourselves of all the benefits that will come. And trusting that our efforts are paying dividends. Because even if they can't be measured, they still count.

 What will convince you that you're not laboring in vain?

July 17

Love your body.

The hard part about doing the postures isn't contorting your body, it's confronting it. I remember a suggestion from a recent class. The teacher said, *When you see yourself in the mirror, stop and enjoy the view.* Consider the weight of those words.

Stop, meaning take the time to confront your truth, without shunning any part of your being.

Enjoy, meaning love yourself enough to live with your physique fully, regardless of size and shape and imperfection.

View, meaning respecting your body as something worth witnessing.

What a difficult thing to do. Because regardless of body type, there isn't a person alive who doesn't cringe a little when staring at his or her body in the mirror. I've been practicing for ten years, and only recently has my inner monologue started to become compassionate toward my body. That's the benefit of daily confrontation. As I learned from the brilliant sex therapist, Chris Donaghue, the best way to increase body esteem is to develop pride through exposure. On the journey to becoming integrated and actualized as human beings, the kindest thing we can do for ourselves is to stop and enjoy the view.

 Are you willing to believe the truth about yourself, no matter how beautiful it is?

July 18

Don't add to your hurt.

Getting sick can be painful. But getting angry and frustrated at ourselves for *being* sick, that can be even worse. It adds an extra layer of suffering on top of our physical ailments. We end up crying not because the stomach bug hurts, but because we think we're the kind of person who shouldn't even have the bug in the first place.

The trick is learning to forgive ourselves when our bodies fail us. Not to become disgusted with our own needs, but to accept and respect ourselves as people who have them. Like when I had a wrist injury and couldn't do yoga for two months. Not practicing wasn't as painful as beating myself up about it was.

 Where in your life do you feel above the situation, as if this should not be happening to you?

July 19

Ignore the critics.

Guru Paramahansa Yogananda said in his bestselling yoga autobiography that his students would be living volumes of his philosophy, proof against the critics.

Time proved him right. The doubters of the world couldn't argue with a generation of people for whom yoga was life-changing. Over one hundred years later, the yoga community still sees criticism—especially for those who practice hot yoga. But those who find that the practice enhances their lives know it doesn't make that much of a difference what others think, as long as it works for them. So let people have their opinions, but stick to the path that is right for you, whether in yoga or elsewhere in life.

 Are you courageous enough to do something critics will criticize?

July 20

Nobody knows how to do life perfectly.

The problem with experts is that they know everything there is to know about what was, but not what could be. In fact, many people kill themselves trying to become experts because they're scared of feeling foolish or looking stupid. Myself included; I spent years surrounding myself with a moat of expertise to protect against the dangers of vulnerability. That's one of the reasons yoga was so attractive to me. Because every class is a beginner's class. There are no experts or geniuses that have it all figured out and know how to do everything perfectly. Even the teachers are still learning. They're guides, not gurus.

Yoga is a practice. It's not what you get after you've done everything right. When you're struggling to touch your elbow to your knee in triangle pose, or when you're fighting to lift both of your legs off the ground in half locust pose, there's no need to beat yourself up for not crushing it. Even if being a perpetual beginner conflicts with the strong and disciplined image you have of yourself.

Part of yoga is letting go of the need to have all our questions answered right away and to expect a quick fix. That's why it's so intimidating. It calls for acceptance of imperfection. And in a world where we spend a lot of time trying to nail everything down, in a culture where we have an obsessive desire to understand everything in our lives, it's a profound relief to let go of the search for the one right way to do things. After all, nobody knows how to do life perfectly. We're all just guessing.

 Are you comfortable being a lifelong beginner?

July 21

Not everything has a finish line.

Our culture is preoccupied with the drama of succeeding and failing. People are constantly setting up binary worlds that allow each other to think in purely win-and-lose terms. That's why we're told over and over that failure isn't an option.

But not everything has a finish line. That's what first attracted me to yoga. It has no end point. It's just wherever you are right now. The girl on the mat next to you might be stronger and thinner and more experienced and has those really cool yoga pants on, but that doesn't make her better and you worse. She's not winning and you're not losing. No dance is out of step. That's why they call it a *practice*.

Krishnamurti said in an interview for *Yoga Journal* that if you are on the right path for you, you will not think in terms of succeeding or failing. It's only when people don't really love what they're doing that they think in those terms. Forget the finish line. Just enjoy practicing.

 Can you give up trying for the podium?

July 22

Give drama a pass.

People overestimate the capacity of human memory. They ascribe far more meaning and drama than needed to the fleeting little conflicts that arise between people, worrying about small interactions and mistakes long after their impact has faded. The reality is, most of the world isn't losing sleep over the person who bumped into them during their commute.

In truth, real life is rarely that dramatic. Most interactions are forgotten, no matter how special and influential we think we are. When we overanalyze our lives, acting as if there were a home audience watching our story unfold, we tend to find intrigue where there is none. We attempt to make stew out of a soup bone.

Thankfully, most people are too busy making their way through their own lives to even think about us. Even when they *are* thinking about us, it's usually just a passing thought. That may be a humbling realization, but the time and energy it saves is worth it.

 Are you giving an insignificant moment more weight than it deserves?

July 23

Ohm is where the heart is.

In yoga, mantras are sacred utterances, sounds, syllables, and words believed to have psychological and spiritual powers. Most familiar is the popular mantra *ohm*. But yoga is also full of more colloquial mantras to keep our postures strong. Here are some mantras, gleaned from teachers, books, audio programs, and posture clinics:

Tighter is lighter. When in doubt, engage muscles. Focus on putting your energy into the parts of your body that feel heavy, and it will be easier to lift your body.

Smooth is fast. Beware of going too strong too soon, or you might tear a muscle and halt your progress. Focus on generating a small amount of pressure and tension first.

Slow is strong. There's zero relationship between speed and success. Take your time getting into and out of the postures. Sixty seconds is much longer than you think.

Less is best. Excessive clothing can hamper mobility. It also adds excess weight and heat to your body during postures. Wear as little as you have to. Your body will thank you. Even if the guy behind you doesn't.

Sweat is sexy. Sweating helps expel toxins, cleanse pores, relieve stress, and kill bacteria. Take it from someone who has been sweat-shamed: It's worth it. Let it flow.

Shaking is shaping. Quivering muscles during difficult poses are a physiological response to working hard. It means your muscles are growing. Just remember to breathe and listen to your body.

 What mantras help protect your practice?

July 24

Open yourself to the swirling air of possibility.

There's a woman at my yoga studio whose water bottle has the following quotation printed on it: Let each moment die its own natural death. Anytime my eyes meet that bottle during class, the words become a bell of awareness for my practice. They remind me that when the pose is over, it's over. Even if my expression of the posture wasn't particularly strong or balanced or precise, I forgive myself for the lapse and move forward into the poetry of the next moment. Fully available to the unknown. Ready to listen to what my body has to say.

Trusting what's happening right now is quite joyful. It lets the next pose in the sequence receive my full attention, a blank slate instead of weighted down by negative expectations. There's no better way to honor yourself in the sequence.

 Do you beat yourself up for not staying in your postures long enough, or do you let go and open yourself to the next moment?

July 25

Our best teacher is often the person who is upsetting us most.

During any given yoga class, there's always at least one person in the room who drives us insane. This individual might be any one of the many yoga personality types, including but not limited to: *dragon breather, space invader, late arriver, phone checker, mat stepper, sweat slinger, chit-chatter.* Or there's my personal favorite, *orgasmic ohm chanter.* It never fails. That person is guaranteed to lay his or her mat down right next to mine. That's why we learn early in our yoga journeys, our best teacher is the person who is upsetting us most.

Patience and forbearance are profoundly difficult to master. But each person who comes into our life, even if it's someone who accidentally elbows our face during a pose, has come to teach us what we need to know. If we allow a stranger in class to shatter our focus, we're the losers missing out on the real benefits of the pose.

If instead we laugh it off and jump back in and learn to accept that very annoyance as our yoga for the day, then we're doing it right. Besides, imagine how many other students *we're* probably annoying in class with *our* own imperfect and unconscious habits.

 Are you ready to be filled with whatever life will teach you?

July 26

Take a step in the direction of faith.

It takes practice to believe in ourselves. That's why it takes weeks, months, and some-times years before our bodies achieve the full expression of certain postures. We need that time to plant the seeds. The genius of yoga is, every day we get onto the mat, we literally step forward as an act of faith in ourselves. That's where belief grows and ability follows.

Balancing stick pose, also known as *tuladandasana*, is the ideal example. It's only ten seconds long, and it's a graceful posture if executed well, especially for us lanky, tall folks. From the side, the body looks like the letter *t*, balanced on one leg. The moment we hear the teacher's command, we have to step forward and make up our mind to use one hundred percent of our strength in half a second. Sometimes, it doesn't quite work out as intended. Perfecting the motion can take many weeks of effort.

But a few months from now, we'll have that one class in which we execute the pose correctly, and the yoga will legitimately change us. Our fragile flame of faith in our muscles and poise is fanned into life. Then nothing will be able to stop us. Just re-member, only the continual act of showing up will build your belief in yourself. If you're not where you want to be in your yoga practice, keep practicing. See if you can push past the part of you that doesn't believe in yourself. Find teachers and fellow students from whom you can borrow courage until you have some of your own. And keep stepping forward as an act of faith in yourself.

 Once you have solid faith in your capabilities, what might be possible for you?

July 27

Rewire your brain.

Yogananda, who first introduced yoga to the Western world back in the 1920s, told his students that repeated performance of any action creates a mental blueprint of subtle electrical pathways in the brain, somewhat like the grooves in a record, and our life follows the grooves that we created in the brain. He believed that the elimination of bad habits could be achieved through contemplation of one's inner consciousness.

Amazingly, Yogananda was talking about neuroplasticity fifty years before doctors even had a word for it. Scientists are just now perfecting the technology to quantitatively prove what the gurus and swamis have been saying for centuries. Maybe that research will finally help dissipate our preconceptions about yoga, and even bring us into a state of discovery that changes us forever.

 When you walk into a yoga room, are you too fixated on your initial judgment that you don't focus on good things while you're there?

July 28

Our own quiet changes are the most convincing statement.

Oda Sessō, the great Zen master, warned that there is little to choose between a man lying in a ditch heavily drunk on rice liquor, and a man heavily drunk on his own enlightenment. I always liked this saying. It's a sobering reminder not to spend too much time preaching from our yoga soapbox.

As much as we love our practice, and as much we're convinced that the world would be a more peaceful place if everyone else practiced too, it's not our job to proselytize everyone we meet into the church of yoga. Nor can we reprogram people's experience banks with positive examples that prove their old yoga assumptions wrong.

Our only job is to put our own mental, physical, and spiritual house in order. Only then, if other people like the view and are curious about the foundation, can we invite them to join us for a class. As my mentor used to say, please don't tell me how to live my life, just love me.

 Are you confident enough to spare people from your yoga zeal?

July 29

Have many paths to happiness.

My favorite spot to practice yoga is close to the mirror, right smack in the middle of the room. I find that having people on both sides of my mat makes me feel connected and supported by the communal energy. It's one of the reasons I practice daily. Yoga gifts me with this profound sense of belonging unlike anything I've ever experienced. Even if it's a hole-in-the-wall studio in a foreign country where I can't understand a word and don't know a soul, it still feels like home.

Conversely, my least favorite spot to practice yoga is in the back corner against the wall. It makes my body feel small and disconnected, and that triggers emotions of loneliness and rejection, sending me back in time to parts of my life where I didn't belong anywhere.

Unfortunately, we don't always have a choice where to set our mats down each time we practice. That's why it's best not to become too attached to any one particular location in the room as our sole vehicle for happiness. Letting go there might just loosen our grip in other places where our attachments are hurting us.

 Where's your favorite spot to practice?

July 30

Practice the posture of patience.

Yoga didn't help me lose weight, but it did help me lose wait. That's something to remember when there are twenty first-time students in the lobby trying to check in at the same time and all you want to do is get into the room and start doing the postures: This is yoga too.

There is no hurry, there are no tests, there is nowhere to get to other than where we are. All we have is right now. Waiting in line to get somewhere is just as important as the place we're getting to. Life *is* the line.

When you meet with frustrations in the line for the dressing room or anywhere else, try this mantra: *This is it, this is as good as it gets, this is the best day of my life.* It's all a matter of perspective.

 What process do you need to own as part of the practice?

July 31

Own your breath, and nobody can steal your peace.

Yoga is a never-ending practice of letting go. It's a ritual of pressing the release valve on ourselves, physically, emotionally, mentally, and spiritually. That's why we begin our series with *pranayama breathing*. This posture teaches us to thread our breath through every action. It reminds us that breath is life. And it shows us that when we own our breath, nobody can steal our peace.

Unfortunately, all of that elevated knowledge goes out the window the minute we don't get our way. Like when our favorite teacher calls in sick. Or when we get stuck practicing behind a clueless first-timer. Or when the room isn't hot enough. Or when the water isn't cold enough. Or when we forget to bring our two-hundred-dollar custom-embroidered, nonslip-surface, ecofriendly, super-absorbent, extra-long yoga mat and have to use one of those gritty studio rentals.

Remember, those moments are part of the yoga too. They may not be postures, but that doesn't mean they're not part of the practice. Just as we let go of our physical imperfections while staring at our half-naked bodies in the mirror, so must we let go of the environmental imperfections that threaten our seamless little yoga nirvanas.

Each time we do so with a return to the breath, the fundamental unit of release. We're all adults. We all know that life doesn't always work out the way we want it to. And unlike spoiled children, yogis don't treat every minor malfunction as a major crisis. We use our lungs to let things go. We breathe in the beauty, breathe out the bullshit.

 Where in your life are you holding your breath?

August 1

Step outside your comfort zone.

I practice yoga with a woman who prescribes homeopathic flower essences. These solutions of brandy and water are petal-infused and supposedly contain the healing properties of that particular plant.

It's pretty far-out stuff. People who sell alternative healing products like flower essences and alkaline water and essential oils can't guarantee remedies for our mental and physical illnesses. What they *can* promise is the power of intention, expectation, and conscious awareness. The ability to improve our overall condition through our attitude. By giving us optimism and a calming ritual, these products ultimately help us feel better. How can we argue with that?

Rather than be quick to judge and label and demonize alternative healing products as spiritual hogwash, the more mature, empathetic, and flexible mindset is to think, hey, any chance people have to positively change the story they tell themselves is worth taking. We all do what we have to do to feel better about ourselves.

We need to recognize that every product is two products in one. There's the thing itself, with its obvious features and benefits. But then there's the related emotional process. The user experience. In many cases, that's what people are really buying. Not what it does, but how they feel when it does it. And that's worth being open to.

 Are you too quick to dismiss things that might be beneficial to you?

August 2

Accept the part of yourself you haven't made peace with.

Most of us have the capacity to be kind and compassionate toward others, but when it comes to looking at ourselves in the mirror, we're much less forgiving. Extending unconditional love for all the parts of ourselves is a terrifying prospect.

Here's one way out of that existential bind. Whenever an undercurrent of self-resentment threatens to hold us in bondage and rob us of peace and joy, blotting out any pleasure we might have had, remember to recite the following mantra: *I love the part of you that…*

Simply look at yourself in the mirror and recite: *I love the part of you that's flabby. I love the part of you that's clumsy. I love the part of you that looks ridiculous in your tight little shorts.* Seven simple words. *I love the part of you that…*

It's an elegant tool for extending unconditional positive regard to all the parts of ourselves.

 Are you still angry at that part of yourself that you haven't made peace with?

August 3

Love your reflection.

Yoga is a place that allows us to accept ourselves fully, even and especially as we may get unflattering glimpses of ourselves. Take spine twisting pose (*ardha matsyendrasana* to you Sanskrit experts). It's the only posture that twists the back from top to bottom. It feels amazing, as spine twisting increases circulation to all the spinal nerves, relieves lower back pain, and helps calm the nervous system.

The only problem is, during this posture, you have to stare at yourself in the mirror from quite possibly the most unflattering angle known to man. The view can include, but isn't limited to, a lovely stomach paunch drooping over the waistband, patches of neck hair sticking out, fat rolls forming into little neck sausages. Not exactly a confidence booster during swimsuit season. Or maybe that's just me.

Although these flaws are exaggerated by the twisting of the body, it's still a painful thing to confront in the mirror. Yet that's the beauty of the practice. Yoga challenges us to see parts of ourselves we have not fully accepted. If we have not made peace with them, seeing how they enable us to execute a posture can help us reach appreciation.

Shakti Gawain's book *Creating True Prosperity* makes a brilliant point about this very experience. She says that life has a way of putting us into situations where we are forced to confront, acknowledge, and develop our disowned selves. Don't avert your eyes. Maybe that's why the mirrors are there: to teach us forgiveness, even from the most unflattering angles.

 What elements of your appearance are you still unwilling to accept?

August 4

Search for the sacred in all things.

Martín Prechtel's book about his experiences apprenticing to a shaman—*The Unlikely Peace at Cuchumaquic*—talks about keeping alive the seeds of our forgotten spiritual side. He says those seeds must be planted and harvested and replanted through various means—not always those you expect. One example his research touches on is a tribe for whom running is a divine act. He writes: *Running was an offering, a feeding of life. And there is no finish line, no heaven-like last act, no glorious arrival. There is only the glorious continuation.*

It's a beautiful way to think about running, and can be translated to yoga. Any good instructor will tell us that for yoga, finishing isn't required, continuing the journey is. Yoga is no race to be competitively won, it's a path to be elegantly followed. That's worth remembering next time we're trying to have the best half-moon pose in class. Focus on the journey to the posture instead of competing over its expression. Inside the pose you may find your own sacred offering.

 Are you playing to win, or playing for the sake of the game?

August 5

Persistence is the great separator.

The last two seconds of most yoga postures are where most students give up. Students figure that half-assing the end of asana won't hurt anyone. But it does hurt themselves. That early exit is representative of an overall attitude of not giving their all.

The most committed students don't just stay in the posture, they push even harder. They know that the only way out is through. Give up before you've reached the finish line, and you lose the benefits.

 Are you persistent in the right places?

August 6

Say "no" to the ego.

No matter how enlightened and accepting we think we are, inside each one of us is a judgmental axe ready to fall. It's difficult to resist. Our ego loves judgment because it gives us a sense of being right and superior. The problem is, it doesn't move us forward. It's just a way of spinning our selfish wheels. It's a waste to occupy ourselves with other people's affairs, gossiping and inventorying and comparing and judging. We must focus on keeping *our* house in order, not theirs. It's like watching the office clock to monitor what time people arrive each morning.

Sarah is always thirty minutes late, and she usually leaves thirty minutes early. Totally unprofessional. Who does she think she is? Somebody should send out a company-wide email and remind all employees that we start work here at nine.

It's exhausting, holding onto these petty little fantasy battles inside our heads. Taking other people's inventories is a pointless endeavor. Besides, we can't learn anything if we're in the judgment business. If that voice shows up, simply say hello and let the judgment continue on its way. Allow others to live their own lives, and you'll have much more time and energy to tend to your own affairs.

 What if the only inventory you needed to take was your own?

August 7

Release your burdens.

Keeping my life as light as possible has become an important goal since I suffered a collapsed lung in my mid-twenties. Now that I know how it feels to be literally crushed under the weight of my own stress, frankly, I'm no longer interested in making each day heavier than it needs to be. I'm no longer in the world domination business.

It's not that I'm against working hard, or that I need to scrub my life clean of any and all effort. But oftentimes, the tasks that weigh us down are rarely as noble as we think. These burdens, heroic as they might seem, are often more trouble than they're worth.

Instead, the goal is for each of us to effect small, concrete ways to make our lives lighter. Like when I noticed that my yoga studio had lockers where I could store my clothes and water bottle overnight, instead of schlepping a stinky backpack to the studio every day. Or when my office installed cloud software for data storage, which meant I no longer had to bring my laptop and hard drives into work each day.

These strategies physically made my life lighter, because I was no longer tethered to my gym bag and briefcase. But they also lightened my emotional load, because I no longer felt the worry of having to manage those extra possessions. It's this strange correlation that happens between the body and the spirit. Once we lay aside the weight that so easily entangles us, we're free to run with endurance the course that is set before us.

 Instead of walking faster, what if you simply carried less in your pack on the trail and then ran?

August 8

Plant an expectation, reap a disappointment.

During our honeymoon in Prague, my wife and I practiced at a local yoga studio, where the instructor said something that I'll never forget: *Try as hard as you like. But expect nothing.*

I probably wasn't ready to understand that idea when I was younger, but it's become my watchword as an adult. I've given up the illusion that I can control anything. I've emptied myself of all expectation and gracefully surrendered to the facts of existence. And I've accepted that just because I spent all that time hoping for a certain outcome, doesn't mean I've earned anything.

If yoga has taught me anything, it's to let everything go and just get on with my life. What a great release and relief.

 What illusions do you cling to?

August 9

Keep evolving.

I love anything that doesn't have a finish line. If there's an endeavor in which you're never done learning and can't possibly have it all figured out, sign me up. That's one of the reasons yoga has become such a centerpiece of my life. There's no finish line. It's a constantly expanding pursuit that makes me feel engaged and tested and stretched.

This concept reminds me of my favorite approach to making passion and intimacy last in our relationships. The Somatica Institute's marriage therapists say that the best part about long-term relationships is that they provide us with an opportunity to grow by forcing us to face our deepest longings and fears as we connect with another human being whose needs, feelings, and desires differ from ours. Getting into a marriage or partnership isn't the end of the line; it's the beginning of a period of conversation and exploration. Relationships aren't stagnant, and neither is a yoga practice. Always seek new ways of experiencing both your partner and your posture.

 How are you growing?

August 10

Keep calm and sweat on.

When the outside world feels like a hot yoga studio, the last thing we want to do is hit the mat and do our postures. But speaking as a man who sweats like a construction worker during even the most mundane activities, summer hot yoga is not as brutal as it sounds. The upside of practicing in warmer months is that the heat of the world starts to bother you less.

Whether it's artificial or natural, regular hot yoga practice trains you to become less bothered by temperature fluctuations than other people. Even if you do sweat through multiple layers of clothing while commuting to work, it's not nearly as sticky and messy as what happens when you're on the mat.

What's more, hot yoga arms you with proper coping tools when the temperature gets too unbearable. Thanks to my practice, vacations in hot climates, steam rooms, and other humid environments are easy to handle. Now I know how to relax through the heat. That's what keeps me coming back to the mat—even in August.

 How do you motivate yourself for hot yoga in the summer when it's sweltering outside?

August 11

Get comfortable with acceptance.

Former Buddhist monk Donald Altman's book *One Minute Mindfulness* reminds us that letting go doesn't mean we don't care, just that we're no longer invested in building a brick wall to try to keep things from changing. It might be a situation at work, or with our family, or with our health; whatever it is, it's out of our hands.

When we let go and accept that we aren't in control, we're not giving up, we're being honest about our situation. Each moment of letting go proclaims to the world, I acknowledge that this is how things are, and although I might want them to be different, I will let go of that belief and allow life to be the way it is.

It's a frustrating practice if you're not used to it and takes years to work through. But it sure beats the alternative. Do you know how exhausting it is to keep denying reality? I'm reminded of when my wrist tendinitis first flared up. I figured the pain would magically go away if I just ignored it. Instead, the pain persisted. I was merely denying reality, not accepting it. The question I had to start asking was: *If I loved myself truly and deeply, would I let myself experience this?*

Of course not. Self-care is not an indulgence. My body is worth taking care of. It was time to stop being such a stoic hero and go get the therapy I needed. That's acceptance. It doesn't mean I like or approve of the situation. Only that I acknowledge reality on reality's terms and take action appropriately.

 How will you widen your capacity for acceptance today?

August 12

Step out of expectation.

The smartest choice I made in my yoga practice was to stop counting. No more looking at the clock. No more head games trying to figure out how much time is left in class. And no more counting how many days in a row I've practiced.

All that quantifying did was create an unnecessary expectation, which started to affect the outcome. The only thing that counts is staying in the moment. The end of a sequence will come whether you anticipate it or not.

 Are you still counting postures?

August 13

Practice aggressive pondering.

Oftentimes when I practice yoga, I set an intention. It's like planting a seed in my brain. I take a particular thought or problem or issue that I'm currently struggling with and use that as a framing device to guide my experience. By the time I'm done, the mental prompt I've layered on top of the rhythmic, repetitive action will produce an insight I wouldn't have discovered otherwise.

Yoga is the ultimate testing ground. The arena where the truth surfaces. Make sure you're using the hot room to its fullest capacity by letting it do that work.

 How will you use your situation as a catalyst to grow and evolve?

August 14

Press the off button.

Stress is a funny thing. It's related to ninety-nine percent of all illnesses, yet it's one of the healthiest tools for motivating us. As long as we keep it in balance, it benefits us, but if it goes too far we'll suffer.

The key to keeping stress from affecting you negatively is learning how to press the off button. Finding a counterweight. Something that creates an inner sanctuary. Something that provides rest, recovery, and renewal to balance out your tension. And something that allows space for quiet within yourself.

Yoga helps with this because the whole point is to gather the quiet so you're able to stand up in the storm. Otherwise, you become so action-oriented that you forget to stop and reflect on what's happening. Stress builds and builds until it overwhelms you. Try stepping back from the urgency instead, and you'll find a better way forward.

 Have you pressed the off button lately?

August 15

Don't presume to judge another person's heart.

Instead of judging others, try to see them as they are. Give them the space to be who they are, instead of molding them into the idealized version of who you want them to be. Honor what's right for them based on their chosen integrity and values, remembering that we would want the same treatment for our own unique journey. At the end of the day, nobody knows what's going on inside anyone else. Everyone is fighting his or her own battle. Even the student practicing next to us in class.

I'm reminded of one of the most famous comics in the world, Eddie Izzard. Izzard loves to tell judgmental people: If you can't handle the fact that I'm a crossdresser, you can go see a therapist and talk to them about *your* problem. It's just fear speaking when we dismiss others. We try to control people's behavior because we cannot control our own anxieties and emotions. But the sad part is, all that does is isolate us further. The easiest way to push people away is to judge them first.

Rather than treat people's choices as problems to be solved, our challenge is to accept those choices as what makes us human and binds us together. Because when we judge, they're not the ones with the issue. We are. The onus is on us.

 Are you seeing people as they are, or as your filters would judge them?

August 16

Be proud of your progress.

Yoga involves falling short, falling out, falling over, falling inward, and pretty much every other kind of falling that you can think of. It can be frustrating and discouraging and occasionally embarrassing, especially if you accidentally kick your neighbor in the face. But enough about my last class.

The important point about falling is, it does not negate the progress you've made. Progress is one of those things that nobody can take away from you. It's imprinted on your cells. So be patient with yourself. Even if your progress is not as rapid as you would like, it's still yours. Forever.

 Where are you willing to fall in your practice?

August 17

~⚬~

Shovelful by shovelful, move forward each time you practice.

The Shawshank Redemption is my favorite movie of all time. It's one of those films that meets you wherever you are, teaching you a new lesson each time you watch it. The prison escape always inspires me. The tunnel out gets dug using nothing but a small rock hammer hidden inside a bible, with the debris brought out into the exercise yard a handful at a time. It wasn't much initially, but the smallest hammer has the capacity to make progress over time through slow, consistent increments.

That process is what yoga is all about. Working slow and hard and progressing shovelful by shovelful, each time you practice. This process is what business is all about too. Speaking from my two decades as an entrepreneur, it wasn't always easy doing things that were not economically rewarding in the instantaneous way I wanted them to be. Focusing on each small step can be frustrating unless you keep an eye on the big picture.

Whatever endeavor you're progressing through, understand that we're all just doing it one handful at a time. If we stay consistent, eventually we'll be able to gaze back and think, wow, look how far we've come.

 Are you taking advantage of compound interest to move forward?

August 18

Respect the group energy.

My biggest struggle in yoga class is staying *with* the class. That's my impatient personality. Rules aren't as appealing as the beat of my own drum. Sometimes that means the class is still in standing separate leg posture trying to touch their foreheads to the floor, and my rebellious spirit tells my body to come out of the pose early and get a drink of water because nobody is gonna tell *me* what to do.

It's a delicate balance between listening to my body and protecting and respecting the group energy. Both are important to a healthy practice.

Fortunately, yoga teaches me to keep my individualistic compulsions at bay. It's really difficult for me. Doing so runs crosswire to the grain of my stubborn soul. But learning to stay with the class is a lesson that pays dividends. I may not like being a team player, but I don't have the right to go it alone just out of contrariness.

 Are you disrespecting the group energy of your community in any way?

August 19

Provide honesty in a way that facilitates growth.

Honesty, although it may hurt someone's ego, will always help that person's practice. My yoga instructor epitomizes this saying brilliantly. She walks the fine line between honestly verbalizing her observations and helping you deepen your practice, without making you feel like a total idiot for screwing up.

For example, instead of telling her students, "If you can't do this posture," she'll say, "If this posture is not available to you." Also, if you fall out of the pose she'll say, "Thank you for listening to your body," as opposed to, "Tall guy! You pathetic worm! Put down that water and get your sweaty ass back onto the mat!"

Honesty shouldn't mean injury. Approach the truth with kindness, not as a weapon. To others, but also to yourself.

 What kind of feedback do you provide others and yourself?

August 20

Be willing to put yourself out of business.

My friend is a chiropractor. In the past five years, he's sent over one hundred of his patients to the yoga studio down the street from his clinic, where he is also a student himself. Sometimes, yoga is the better course of treatment for their ailments.

The other day his assistant yelled at him for sending too much business away out of fear the patients would fall in love with yoga and never come back for another adjustment again. But as a true professional, a true artist, and a true champion of human health, my chiropractor friend told his assistant that a good doctor tells his patients, "I hope you never have to come in here again."

That's the path that creates loyalty by showcasing integrity. It also acknowledges that each situation is unique and requires different treatment. Make sure that those you rely on for care in your own life take a similar approach.

 How are you putting the needs of others first?

August 21

Do the drishti.

It's tempting to let our eyes wander during yoga class. Especially when we're practicing next to veteran students whose taut bodies move gracefully like swans across the water.

That's why teachers will suggest we find a point on the wall, a crack in the ceiling, or a strand in the carpet and use it as our single point of vision. It's called *drishti gaze*, which is a consciously directed, unwavering, steady, and detached focus. Not only does it help us stay balanced and present in our postures, but it also helps relax the mind. After all, most of our sensory input enters the body through the eyes.

Fluttering our gaze around the yoga room like a hummingbird only forces our brain to process more information and stimuli. It's distracting. When we look at one thing and hold our gaze gently, the hamster wheel inside our head slows down. Quiet eyes, peaceful mind.

 How has yoga transformed your vision?

August 22

Calm the monster inside your head.

Parkinson's law states that work expands to fill the time available for its completion. In other words, if we have a problem, we will use all of the time available to obsess over it. There simply aren't enough structures and constraints to keep our minds occupied. That goes for personal issues or for work tasks, especially if we freelance or otherwise set our own schedule.

Unlike people working a more traditional career path, complete with bosses and employees and offices and performance reviews, we can end up spending our entire morning walking a hole in the carpet. That's one of the reasons yoga has been so transformative for me. As a writer, I spend all day living inside my head. It's in the job description.

Yoga is a release from that. When I walk into the studio for those critical ninety minutes, all I can do is focus on my breathing and pay exquisite attention to my body. It's too hot and too crowded and too intense to drift off inside my head. By the time class is over, every problem I walked into the room with has been washed away.

We all run the risk of having too much freedom. Too much time to reflect and obsess and disappear down the rabbit hole of our own mythology. If the familiar clouds start to gather above your head, give that energy something else to do. Give it a hot room to practice in.

 What will you do when you get tired of beating your head against a brick wall?

August 23

Reality never changes—we do.

There was a guy at our studio who did yoga every single day for three consecutive years. His surgeon had suggested it as part of his rehabilitation program after he had suffered a catastrophic motorcycle accident. And so, he came to class every day, with both arms on crutches, worked harder than anybody, and the smile never left his face.

He was truly inspiring. Practicing next to him made our postures better by way of osmosis. One night I asked him if yoga was helpful for pain management. And he said that although he was not free of pain, yoga *did* give him more positive ways to handle it.

That's the mindset each of us should strive for. Instead of finding ample ways to deny every unpleasant feeling we have, we equip ourselves with the tools to manage whatever arises. Because reality never changes, only our acceptance of it does.

 What setback are you ready to smile at?

August 24

Accept where you are right now.

There are six heating ducts in our yoga studio. They're crucial for getting the room temperature over one hundred degrees. But if you can avoid practicing directly under them, it's for the better. Because that hot air blowing directly on your face during camel pose can burn your fingers a bit during vertical stretching poses.

Keep in mind, though, the yoga room is a larger metaphor for life. And so, sometimes it's a crowded weekend morning and you're running late and there's only one spot left on the floor and you have no choice but to practice under the heating duct. There's no running from it.

Despite that, some frustrated students will move their mat two and three times to various spots around the room during class, denying reality like it's their job. They desperately seek a spot that meets their heat requirements. But that's not yoga. The goal is to meet yourself where you are, physically, emotionally, spiritually, and spatially.

 Are the things you dislike really unendurable?

August 25

Regulate your compulsion to control.

Hot yoga is meditative and peaceful and connected and expressive. It's also messy and sweaty and crowded and imperfect. That's a good thing. The nature of the practice regulates our compulsion to control, manage, neaten, organize, and label ourselves. It also helps us regulate our compulsion to control, manage, neaten, organize, and label the lives of others.

In my first few months of yoga, I could literally feel the controlling instinct welling up inside of me during each pose. *Must fix mat. Must wipe sweat. Must straighten towel. Must help the guy practicing next to me do the postures correctly.* That's the codependent's creed. What else can I do for you to make *me* more comfortable?

Soon enough, the yoga helped me accept people and situations as they were, instead of as I would have liked them to be. And that was huge. On and off the mat. Each of those micro-moments of acceptance during the postures seeped into the rest of my life. They stopped me from subtly controlling and molding everyone I met into my own image. The best part is, when we trust the natural flow of our experiences instead of trying to control everything, we experience less pain and greater joy.

 How has yoga transformed your compulsion to control?

August 26

Relax and soak up everything you came here to give yourself.

Savasana, also known as "corpse pose," is the most anatomically neutral yoga position. It reduces stress and fatigue on muscles and joints. It also helps lower blood pressure, slow respiration, and reduce heart rate. Most teachers say it's the most important posture of the practice.

Despite how easy it looks, it's profoundly challenging. The only thing savasana requires of you is to simply *be*. To take a ride on your sweat instead of trying to wipe it off. As my teacher loves to say, *relax and soak up everything you came to class to give yourself*. The best part of savasana is that its basic principles can also be applied to life off the mat. It's all about putting yourself in a neutral position. Not necessarily physically, but mentally, emotionally, and spiritually.

I recently traveled to Malaysia to deliver a presentation. Malaysia was one of the most colorful, friendly, juicy countries I ever visited. The audience was engaged, the food was spicy, and the weather felt like I had never left yoga class. What I loved most about the experience was that it sent my mind to a neutral position. Because when you're swimming in a waterfall in the middle of the jungle ten thousand miles away from home, with no cell phone or contact with the outside world, your inner life suddenly gets very clear and very quiet. Like taking a mental savasana. Not surprisingly, by the time we returned home, I felt completely rejuvenated. Like I had just finished a seven-day yoga class. Dead body pose? Perhaps. But true savasana is when you feel most alive and immersed in the moment.

 What's your favorite posture?

August 27

Relax into your yoga reality.

If there's one thing yoga teaches us, it's that our body produces symptoms that demand attention. When we don't pay them heed, we pay the price.

Yoga has become my workout, my meditation, my service, my organizing principle, and my social circle, to name a few. It's hard to let go of practicing some days because it's so important to my life. But when the body speaks, I listen. Otherwise I injure myself.

That means that if there is a back problem or a flu virus or some other bodily issue that needs addressing, I don't go anywhere near the studio. That hurts too, but only for a day. What's more important is that my symptoms are clues to something inside of me that needs work. Even if that work doesn't include practicing yoga, it's my duty to address it. Stepping away from the postures briefly can be yoga too.

 How are you compassionate to your body?

August 28

Relaxation is a second full-time job.

If we're lucky enough to reach a state of complete relaxation in which we feel unburdened by life's troubles, it's probably not because we somehow mastered mindfulness or meditated enough or practiced yoga for ninety days straight. It's likely because we acknowledged, accepted, erected, and protected our own boundaries. That's where true relaxation comes from. Living a life with limits.

Back in my workaholic days, when my life had about as many boundaries as a hyperactive toddler, relaxing didn't exist for me. My home wasn't a haven for respite and human connection, it was an extension of the workplace. On any given day or night, I would find myself either completely overwhelmed by work, or in withdrawal from it. The minute you walked into the house, *kablam*, you were punched in the face with the circus known as my career.

There was no room for non-work pursuits. There was no physical or psychological distance between work and everything else. As my therapist used to joke, *you were either in my work, or in my way*. There were no cognitive boundaries either. My attention was perpetually held hostage by work.

True relaxation is something that comes from having boundaries that are airtight and completely integrated into your life. Don't have that? Time to get your own boundaries. Erect them. And protect them. This process requires persistent, dedicated effort. But it's worthwhile in trying to protect you from yourself.

 Where in life do you feel the need for more effective boundaries?

August 29

Rely on your intuitive faculties.

Sometimes serving yourself better requires getting quiet and listening for your own inner voice to guide you. This is easier said than done, of course. In my experience, the best practice for doing so is to put yourself in situations that demand total presence.

Personally, I use yoga. The total presence allows you to stop and listen to the voice of your true self. Even if you don't like what it has to say, you listen anyway. After all, listening is a form of loving. Scientist/inventor George Washington Carver said it best: There is nothing that will not give up its secrets if you love it enough.

 How will you be loving today?

August 30

Respect the paradox of the journey.

As a student of yoga you have to achieve balance between total relaxation and complete exertion. A helpful way of doing so is to ask two simple questions:

Where can you afford to be patient? Not idle, not passive, but patient. Because as long as you don't wait so long that it becomes too late to take action, and as long as you're not investing valuable time waiting for something that's never going to happen, it usually pays to wait it out.

Where can you allow yourself to be impatient? Not reckless, not irresponsible, but impatient. Although patience is a virtue, impatience pays the mortgage. Sometimes you just have to trust yourself, trust the process, and gather whatever momentum you can to start moving in the right direction.

Knowing the answer that's right for your particular situation? That just takes knowing yourself.

 How can you be patient and impatient simultaneously?

August 31

Go inch-by-inch.

Yoga is a practice of inches. Every day that we hit the mat, we must discipline ourselves in a thousand micro-moments. Sometimes class is one long exercise in restraint. I have to resist the urge to grunt, breathe dramatically, fidget my limbs, fix the towel, tighten the muscles on my forehead, look around the room at other students, stick my hands on my hips like a yoga diva, and, of course, glare at the teacher when she holds postures just a little too long.

Sound like a frustrating ninety minutes? Perhaps. But that was my yoga for the day. Because I know that as I begin to be disciplined in these small ways, the bigger tests of my discipline will become much easier to handle.

Hartley Coleridge, son of legendary poet Samuel Taylor Coleridge, was right when he observed, *If we take care of the inches, we will not have to worry about the miles.* That's how the discipline of yoga works. We focus on small victories. Micro-improvements. Subtle corrections that amass a solid foundation from which real growth occurs. If I can resist the urge to wipe a drop of sweat in between postures today, then maybe I can execute a full inversion in the posture tomorrow.

 How many small victories did you accomplish today?

September 1

Trust that daylight always comes back.

Fear has a lot of shady disguises. When I attempt a new or difficult posture, fear masquerades as the voice of wisdom and reason. It tricks me into believing that I'm in greater danger than I really am, and that I'd better back away from taking any risks. It's so hard not to listen.

But the thing fear doesn't want us to know is, it has limited stamina. It may be fast off the starting blocks, but it rarely stays alive for the long game. If we're willing to be patient and sit through that initial panic, we can wait it out. Fantasy author Neil Gaiman's popular essay on the power of ghost stories, "Ghost in the Machine," said it best: *Fear is a wonderful thing, in small doses. You ride the ghost train into the darkness, knowing that eventually the doors will open and you will step out into the daylight once again.*

That's how fear works. Like a weather pattern. It has a beginning, a middle, and an end. And if we learn to wait out the storm, maybe even dance in its puddles from time to time, we should be okay.

 How do you handle the fear that sets its mark on your life?

September 2

Create your own rituals.

When we want to send a message to ourselves or a higher power, ritual is an amazing conduit. It might be part of your practice, it might be part of your commute or bedtime routine; choose the time of day that speaks to you. Here's how rituals work:

First, they communicate to you that you're worth giving this moment to.

Second, they communicate to the divine that you're willing to honor the beauty of the present moment.

Third, they communicate to other people that they're worth pausing for.

Fourth, they communicate to the world that it's worth slowing down and paying attention to.

The built-in rituals are what first attracted me to yoga. The practice of *namaste*, whose meaning is "the spirit in me honors the spirit in you," is exactly what you communicate when you ritualize your life. Honor, spirit, and respect. Even if nobody notices but you, the accumulation of those daily rituals will slowly bring a deeper significance into your life.

 Can you honor your spirit today?

September 3

Safety and security are two different things.

Bikram constantly reminds us that if you own your breath, nobody can steal your peace. This isn't only yoga advice; it's life advice. No matter how unsafe the surrounding world is, when you thread your breath (or *prana*) through every move you make, nobody can shatter the rock that is your foundation.

Prana imposes form on the chaos of the world. Your breath becomes your security, even when the world around you feels unsafe. When you get stuck, your lungs are your lifelines. I urge you to take a breath, even if you don't think you need one.

 How can your breath become your security amid the chaos of the world?

September 4

Avoid other people's drama.

In any given yoga class, there are a thousand potential distractions. Loud noises, flickering lights, annoying voices, blasting heaters, and sweaty puddles, just to name a few. But let us never underestimate the most distracting thing of all: *other people's drama and conflict.*

We can count on it in almost every class. The student next to you might start frantically rubbing out a cramp, huffing under her breath at the teacher, or, my personal favorite, obsessively checking incoming messages on her smart watch.

We mustn't allow these moments to throw us off course. It's so hard, especially when we're not feeling particularly confident about our own practice. We can get seduced into taking other people's yoga inventories, but we should be focusing on our breath. They can handle themselves, just as we need to only focus inward.

 What's your biggest distraction during class?

September 5

See what body you have today.

Many promises are attached to yoga. People start taking class for any number of reasons, from healing their bodies to calming their minds to finding their second spouse. But as with most things in life, nobody gets exactly what they thought they were going to get. Especially on the mat. Ask anyone who's practiced for more than a few months. The benefits of yoga are many, but they are often not what we thought. Walk into the room, see what body you have today, and tune into whatever it wants to teach you. Here are several of the unexpected gifts my practice gave me:

Yoga didn't make me stronger, but it did strengthen my capacity to meet the requirements of living.

Yoga didn't help me shed weight, but it did help me accept and even love the parts of my body that were carrying a few extra pounds.

Yoga didn't turn my arms into registered weapons, but it did help me build the invaluable muscle of stillness.

 When was the last time you got exactly what you expected?

September 6

See yourself in a different light.

When I practice at local studios on my travels, there's instant community. In any city we visit, the people welcome us as fellow students, seekers, and supporters of this practice. Many times we bump into old yoga friends, friends of friends, or even instructors who did their teacher-training with people from our home studio. It's magical. We never know who we might meet. Including ourselves.

That's the other cool thing about practicing at different studios. We quite literally see ourselves in a different light. At our home studio, we tend to stick to our yoga routines. Practicing in the same locations each time. Sitting out the same poses each time. But at a new studio with different lighting, different mirrors, different traditions, different floors, different people, different water, and different heat and humidity, we find different vantage points from which to observe who we are.

Yoga seeks to give us a new sense of identity by enlarging our inner horizon. Traveling this week? Get out into the community and press the flesh with the local yogis. They will help you see yourself anew.

 What habits are preventing you from making progress toward becoming the best version of yourself?

September 7

Show people they've already achieved victory.

Whenever new students come to practice at my yoga studio, I always make it a point to congratulate them in the locker room for sticking it out the whole ninety minutes.

At least you stayed in the room the whole time. I've been here for years and not all first-timers do. Consider that a victory.

Every time I've said this, new students never fail to become energized. Many of them even come back. Amazing what a little encouragement will do, how easy it is to give—and how too often, we don't make the time.

 What could you say to someone to reinforce their self-belief?

September 8

Sign up for a series of choices and challenges.

Each yoga posture is filled with small opportunities for us to challenge ourselves. From the physical challenge of keeping our weight in our heels, to the emotional challenge of forgiving ourselves when we fall out of posture, to the social challenge of joining the communal yoga experience, to the mental challenge of keeping our eyes on our own mat and not on that hunky rugby player in the front row.

When we walk into the yoga room, the goal isn't to dread the hard postures and look forward to the easy ones. It's to meet each pose as an opportunity to explore our strengths and flexibility. Here's a fun exercise my yoga buddies often do in the locker room after class. We ask each other: *What's your least favorite posture right now?*

Our answers are always changing, because we're always changing. To practice yoga is to sign up for a series of choices and challenges, and to relish each one.

 How are you mindfully being part of your process of change?

September 9

Simplify your transitions, save your energy.

One of the first lessons I learned as a songwriter was, *The music is not in the notes, but in the space between them.* Yoga works similarly. What we do when we're not holding the postures is an equally important element of the practice. That's yoga, too. Even in that brief moment between camel pose and rabbit pose, for example, there is still wisdom to be gained.

My frequent yoga teacher, Channing, reminds us to simplify our transitions. To save our energy for the postures, instead of burning useless calories fixing our hair or walking dramatic circles around our mats. By choosing stillness and simplicity instead, we create space rather than noise. In that quiet, you never know what you might hear.

 Are you learning from the moments between poses?

September 10

Don't slide into complacency.

Addiction of any sort isn't a state of mind that wears off over time, but a permanent change in the shape and chemistry of the brain. Unfortunately, it's more common than many realize. If you're counting your sober days, months, or even years, your time free of an eating disorder, or downward spiral, don't forget to watch your step. You may have walked a long way since you began, but the monkey you pulled off your back has been keeping pace with you the entire way. Knowing that the darkness you already worked so hard to free yourself from can return at any time? God help us.

That's why we have to be vigilant. Not necessarily about drugs, but about all of the behaviors and habits and obsessions that threaten to steal our peace. Because the body never forgets. Take stress, for example. During the more chaotic chapters of life, it's easy to reach a point where it's so familiar, we take it for granted. We write it off and compartmentalize it and think to ourselves, I guess that's just how it is.

When our guard is down or we get so arrogant that we think ourselves unsinkable is precisely when the darkness strikes. In the words of one of my instructors: *Don't get complacent in your practice. Fear will sniff it out and come back to beat you in the next pose.* She's right. Calamity will shake up whatever we have come to assume was permanent, unless we remain on our guard. The monkey mind is always looking for an easy way to calm itself. Use your yoga to make sure the healthy antidote, not the destructive one, predominates.

 Is your success delivering you into a wilderness of false assumptions and bad habits?

September 11

Smash all the rules, simply by breathing.

I once heard my yoga teacher say that the less breath you feed your fear, the bigger your fear gets. Whether you're on the mat or out in the world, as soon as you see the warning signs that you are getting into a crisis or losing control, just breathe.

Three easy steps. Inhale, pause, exhale. Then repeat. Even if it does sound like something a preschool teacher would tell an upset student who's holding her breath until she passes out on the floor, breathing is a highly underrated emotional tool. Simply being able to breathe means being in control, albeit in a small form, and is often enough to carry you through the moment.

That's the beautiful thing about the breath. It doesn't need to be told what to do. The goal is to get to the point where the breath is breathing you, not the other way around. Next time life gets a little too overwhelming, use your lungs to make a bridge away from fear and anxiety.

 When was the last time you successfully breathed through something difficult?

September 12

Reap what your body sows.

Fall is my favorite season. Crisp air, falling leaves, and of course, warm caramel-flavored drinks at the local coffee shop. It's the season of transformation, when all the hard work we've put in pays off. We reap our yoga harvest. We finally stand on one leg or touch our forehead to the ground.

There's something deeply nourishing in gathering the fruit of our labors. Fall reminds us that our faith and patience will pay off in due time. We must wait for our crops to ripen before we attempt to collect them. The season teaches us to trust in the natural progression of things.

 What harvest are you ready to gather?

September 13

Shed your outer layer.

The advantage of doing yoga in the evening is that you can leave any accrued burdens on the mat. Whatever physical and emotional grime accumulated throughout the day, we can release ourselves from it all.

Not unlike journaling, yoga is a method to purge everything that happens to us. It might be stress from our relationships or work, or it might literally be dirt from our toil and efforts, whether it comes from working outside, being involved in play with our kids, or just being outside running our errands.

Personally, one of the most satisfying moments of my yoga is when I look down at my towel and notice that my footprints have left marks on the fabric. Twin sacred divine dirt clods. Physical manifestations of the day's work dripping off of me. Proof that my body, mind, and soul have been cleansed. I left it all on the mat.

 What other outlet helps you purge everything that happens to you?

September 14

Start from a place of commonality.

Sociologists say that the three conditions crucial to making close friends are proximity, repeated unplanned interactions, and a setting that encourages people to let their guard down and confide in each other. That comes naturally when you're in college, but when you're older, friendship is a different story. After a certain age, making new friends is hard. We don't have the luxury of proximity we did in college. People end up wrapped up in their career and family.

But although making friends as an adult is difficult, it's not impossible. The secret is finding centers of belonging to do the heavy lifting for you. Yoga studios are an ideal tool for doing so. The goal is to find a sanctioned organization of which you can become an engaged member. Relationships flourish when they start from a place of shared values. This doesn't mean you should only befriend mirror images of yourself. But when you seek out people who have overlapping value systems, when you repeatedly connect with individuals who choose to make meaning in similar ways, most of the heavy lifting is already done for you. Now all you have to do is go deeper.

One of the micro-practices I find useful in striking up new acquaintances is reciprocal disclosure. I try to learn one new fact about each person at my yoga studio each time we meet, while also revealing one new fact about myself. This fosters intimacy, uncovers new points of connection, and deepens the relationship. We never know what the people around us might have to offer until we reach out to ask.

 What are your centers of belonging?

September 15

Start small and the path will illuminate itself.

For the first few years of my yoga practice, there were certain postures I didn't even attempt. They just seemed too advanced for a beginner like me. Until one day when my yoga friend said something I'll never forget: We don't always need to get better, just less threatened.

A few minutes later, our class came to the dreaded camel pose. The backbending posture that opens the entire front side of the body. The mother of all yogic movements. Thanks to my friend's insight, for the first time in my yoga life, instead of sitting out on my mat and watching the other students in admiration, I decided to give it a shot. I inhaled, leaned back, and before I knew it, I had achieved the full expression of the posture. I couldn't believe my own body. And the surprising part was that executing the pose wasn't nearly as scary as I imagined. Not even close. In fact, by the time the posture was finished, I thought to myself, that was it? That's what I was scared of for two years?

Turns out, competence wasn't the issue, confidence was. I allowed fear to have too loud a voice. But the minute I actually paid attention to the man behind the curtain, everything changed. That's the thing about fear. When the voice doesn't scare us, when the reputation doesn't intimidate us, and when the smoke doesn't dissuade us, we become the great and powerful ones.

 How will you recognize and remove the resistance that inhibits you?

September 16

Stay in the room.

If the hardest part about practicing yoga is getting to the hot room, the second-hardest part is staying there, both literally and figuratively. Teachers tell students to stay in the room because, in physical terms, it's just good yoga etiquette. The act of stepping off of the mat and tiptoeing around other people's space can be distracting, disrespectful, and sometimes even dangerous.

Mentally staying put can be a little tougher to enforce on yourself. You may intend not to spend the entire class planning out your dinner or rifling through your to-do list for the rest of the weekend, but it's easy for our minds to drift off our mats. We can be physically in the practice without being present to our surroundings.

I struggle with this version of staying in the room on a weekly basis, to the point that I will start performing the wrong posture and not even realize it until I snap out of fantasyland and notice that I'm the only student still standing up. Whoops. All you can do is laugh, let yourself off the hook, and remember that it's only yoga and nobody's even paying attention to you anyway. Then bring your attention back to the mat and try to keep it there.

So keep your body and your brain in the room. I know it's tempting to step out, but unless it's a true emergency, you'll be better off staying present. Everything you came for is waiting for you on the mat.

 What mental obstacles are keeping you from being present?

September 17

Pay attention to the lessons that won't leave you alone.

We're told that when the student is ready, the teacher will appear. But what we're not told is that if we *don't* learn the lesson, the teacher will come back.

My yoga practice is quite impatient. I will enter and exit postures according to my own schedule. There's no doubt that my rebellious and individualistic tendency to march to the beat of my own drum drives my instructors crazy. Thankfully, as highly trained and deeply experienced teachers, they accept my unwillingness to learn my lesson. Instead, they keep reminding me. John, one of our alumni teachers, always nailed me: "Scott, stay with the rest of the class. Scott, don't come out early. Scott, move with the words."

These corrections bother me at a visceral level. They trigger childhood memories of teachers, parents, and other authority figures scolding me for not being a team player and refusing to follow the herd, and it pains me every time. But that's yoga. That's life. That's everything. Until the lesson is finally learned, the teacher is going to keep coming back. And back. And back. Until maybe we realize it has something to tell us.

 What lesson are you pretending not to need to learn?

September 18

Stillness is the water that washes down the pill.

Ever tried taking a pill without water? It's dreadful. The medication gets stuck in the back of your throat and leaves that nasty, chalky chemical taste in your mouth. *Blech.* Taking a pill without water can cause tissue damage and obstruction or inflammation of the esophagus. There's even a name for it: *pill-induced esophagitis.* Of course, all of this can be avoided by simply drinking the right amount of water when taking your medication.

What does this have to do with yoga? Everything. Because if you want to receive the mental, physical, and spiritual benefits of the practice, you need an aid to make the medicine go down. And we're not talking about water here. That's why our instructor reminded us during a recent class: Stillness is the water that washes down the pill. Only when we truly relax and stop fidgeting (mentally as well as physically) can we soak up all the benefits we came to class to receive.

 Do you need more still water, or more stillness?

September 19

Treat others with compassion.

When you interact with a friend's baby and it suddenly starts crying, no one takes it personally. You don't get all defensive and suspicious and cynical, ruminating to yourself, *Man, that baby is out to get me. Little punk doesn't know who he's dealing with.* Instead, you simply look for the benevolent, human explanations for the child's behavior. He must be hungry or cold or tired or restless or wants his mommy or needs to poop. How precious.

Meanwhile, when we're in the locker room after class and the new student suddenly starts acting in a way that's surprising or bizarre, all of our patience, kindness, and humility go out the window. We forget the fact that everybody we meet is carrying a heavy burden. We forget the fact that we never know what's going on in people's lives when we encounter them, and we plunge headfirst into the judgment vortex.

A smarter move is to flex the muscle of compassion. To look at that person lovingly and think, *Wow, I wonder what transitions he might be facing right now. I wonder what emotional continuum she might be negotiating today.* Issues like these are the adult version of having a poopy diaper. Remembering that it's probably not about us can help us meet more and more of our interactions with kindness and understanding.

 Are people truly out to get you, or are they just tired, hungry, or restless?

September 20

Surrender to the itch and just let it tickle you.

Accepting that not all battles can be won, or are worth the time and energy to fight, frees up millions of potential calories for more useful things. Sometimes, it's best to just give up. My yoga practice has strengthened my muscle of surrender.

It's important to practice this one, because most people have no frame of reference for surrender. Especially men. We are taught that surrender is a word for losers and weaklings. The social cost of total surrender for us is high due to those social pressures. But in the past ten years, my ability to let things go has skyrocketed. My teacher sees me fidgeting in between the postures every day. She reminds me: Surrender to the itch and just let it tickle you. Here are a few of my favorite white flag moments:

Surrendering my sense of drama, knowing that the person practicing next to me is not going to confront me in the hallway after class for sweating too much.

Surrendering my sense of urgency, trusting that I will still make it to work on time, even if I do take an extra few minutes in final savasana.

Surrendering my digital tethers at the door, remembering that there are only two people who call me anyway, and one of them is practicing right next to me.

The cool part is, surrender is only the beginning. Because once we surrender, we then get to live in the new peace we have found. It's glorious. In surrendering to life as it unfolds, we find ourselves on a great adventure.

 On what imaginary battles are you wasting valuable creative energy?

September 21

Surround yourself with inspiring mentors.

When I started practicing hot yoga, I was a beginner in every sense of the word. I'd never done it before, never even wanted to do it, and certainly never thought I'd actually do it. Especially since I heard the classes involved ninety minutes in a hot, humid room. I told as much to my instructor the first time I walked into the studio. She smiled and replied, Yeah, that's what I said thirteen years ago. More amazingly, she still kept the spirit of a beginner despite her experience.

Now, here I am, practicing every day. Why? Because I initially surrounded myself with veteran starters. People who renewed their enthusiasm and commitment as time went on. These are the people who will fuel your ability to execute. Find mentors and friends who invigorate you to follow in their footsteps.

 Who do you take inspiration from?

September 22

Sweat is holy water.

At my studio, there are people we see every single day. We know their names, we memorize their tattoos, we give them friendly nods at the beginning of class, and we chat them up in the locker room to talk about our respective practices. In many cases, that's the extent of our relationship. Casual acquaintances. Meditation buddies. Recreational companions. Fellow members of the community.

But the beautiful part is, even though we may not know one another on a social or professional level, we still understand and sympathize with and love each other as women and men journeying together on the road to wellness. After all, we're all in this together. Yogis sweat together, we struggle together, and we grow our inner spirits together. It creates a unique form of intimacy that can't be found anywhere else. Perhaps it's time for a new bumper sticker: The community that perspires together, inspires together.

 Is that sweat coming out of your pores, or is it holy water?

September 23

Build your foundation.

If you're losing your balance, struggling to execute, and feeling unclear about what the next step is, the smartest, easiest, and most effective strategy is to engage your core. Activating the midsection muscles always creates a foundation from which any posture can grow. No matter how long you've been practicing, no matter what injuries you walk into the room with, you can't go wrong when you emphasize your core. If you did nothing else for the entire class but focus on that, you'd still receive the benefits of the poses. When in doubt, engage your core.

This principle isn't just helpful in the yoga room. It's also a helpful strategy for taking action off the mat. Doubt is an unavoidable feature of the human landscape, and to soldier through, we need to be rooted. The secret in executing anything is having that default move ready to go. That way, when the doubt comes crashing in, we don't have to think or ponder or choose. We simply engage our core. Do that, and you'll be able to start from a strong position, every time.

 What default move helps overcome your feelings of doubt?

September 24

Be open to the unexpected.

The other day our yoga teacher called in sick at the last minute. By the time I got to the studio, fifteen annoyed students were standing in the lobby, looking at their cell phones, wondering if anybody was going to show up. It was hot. It was dark. It was seven in the morning. I called the owner, but nobody responded. I waited a few minutes and called again. Nothing. The clock was ticking. Nobody was interested in missing their daily practice, including me, and the top of the hour was rapidly approaching. Somebody had to do something.

Okay everybody, here's the deal, I announced. *Don't worry about signing in. Class is free today. Just lay down your mats, grab your towels, and head inside. We're starting in two minutes.* I changed clothes, grabbed my laptop, and walked into the room. Located the audio version of the yoga series I often listen to when I travel. Turned the volume to eleven, set the computer down in the middle of the carpet, and started class. And. Everything. Went. Perfectly. We had a great practice. Finished right on time. Nobody was late for work. I even got a nice round of applause after final savasana.

Except from this one guy. He was so infuriated that there wasn't a real instructor, he walked out of the room five minutes into class. The moral of the story is, flexibility is only fifty percent physical.

 How will you be flexible today?

September 25

Take extreme ownership over your practice.

Barack Obama's legendary speech from his first presidential campaign popularized the phrase *We are the ones we've been waiting for.* In the yoga world, that saying inspires me daily to double down on my sense of personal responsibility. To take extreme ownership over my yoga practice, never waiting for some external process to start working its magic.

That's what I love about the postures. They're portable. Yoga requires no equipment beyond the readiness to practice it. You can do the postures on the beach, in a hotel room, or in the backyard. You can watch videos online, you can listen to audio recordings, or you can choose a sequence of your own favorite postures from memory.

Sure, going to a yoga studio with a trained instructor is nice, but it's not necessary. It's like that moment in the third act of the fantasy movie when the protagonists suddenly realize that they don't need some magic ring or fancy weapon to access their powers. The power is already inside of them. It always was.

 Are you ready to be your own savior?

September 26

Take responsibility for your own realizations.

Yogananda said that yoga is a practice that contains timeless truths that can reorient our very nature. During yoga, he was wholeheartedly listening to himself, but, not bound by his limited identity, able to access the reservoir of cosmic energy.

Sounds like an inspiring experience. But although yoga can rejuvenate our nature, we have to allow it to first. That's a practice in and of itself. It takes conscious effort to develop one's spiritual muscles.

Often this happens via meditation, but it can also be done by the simple act of journaling. I once visited a studio that had a blank notebook stationed in the lobby for students to share their epiphanies, insights, and other visions received during class. Some entries were single words, some were drawings, some were only a few short sentences, and others were half-page gushings documenting the wisdom received during class. No matter the format, all of the entries were setting the writer on his or her own path of self-discovery. Sometimes, the first step is just to pay attention to our realizations, noting what causes us to vibrate on a higher level.

 Are you willing to hear what your journey is telling you?

September 27

Take the calm with you.

Finding peace in yoga class is a worthwhile goal that millions of people hope to accomplish every day. The true test, however, is when you learn to transfer those feelings to the rest of your life. *Take the calm with you*, as it were. It's harder than it sounds, and it often happens without our conscious awareness. When you walk out of the hot room feeling calm and relaxed, remember to take that calm with you. Because whatever work you do during class, it's all prologue to the real postures that lay ahead.

Here's how the story usually goes when people start practicing yoga regularly: After a few months or years, something shifts inside them. Their stress level has plummeted. Their pain tolerance has increased. They don't get road rage anymore. Mistakes and failures at work roll off their back. Petty little battles with friends and family that used to make their blood boil no longer activate their anger. The list goes on and on. The improvements happen not because people specifically tried to improve in those particular areas, but because yoga acted as a force multiplier to make them more even-keeled.

 Are you taking radical responsibility for the energy you bring to the world?

September 28

Take your anger and make it awareness.

The goal of this practice is not perfecting mindfulness or levitating yourself into a meditating pretzel, but rather creating an enlarged awareness of your bodily sensations. It's about enlivening and engaging muscles you didn't know you had and noticing and naming feelings you didn't realize were there.

Each of these experiences gives you power to push to new heights of awareness. That's how you know the yoga is working. Not just when you start touching your head to your knee, but also when you stop bristling with impatience towards life's trivial irritants. Not just when you learn to flex your inner thigh muscle to balance, but also when you take your anger and productively put it into your legs instead of eating three slices of pizza in five minutes.

That's awareness. It's the state of consciousness that frees you from reactivity and the muscle that gives you the power to step out of frustrating patterns and into renewal.

 Does your anger belong in an asana?

September 29

Stop anticipating.

Don't anticipate your instructor's words. Stay in the now. Stop thinking about what movement is coming next. Wait until the instructor says so to come out of your posture. Quitting early, even by half a second, sacrifices your integrity and shows disrespect to your fellow yogis.

One of the major blocks to effective listening is anticipating. We too often hold conversations focused only on getting our piece in, rather than receiving what our friend or colleague has to tell us. Anticipating what we're going to say next consumes us. We may even anticipate (wrongly) what the person we're speaking with is going to say, all in the service of planning how we're going to prove the other person wrong or add our own anecdote. Chances are, not much connection comes out of those interactions. In yoga as in life, we don't benefit by looking ahead. Let yourself just be in the moment.

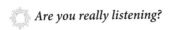 *Are you really listening?*

September 30

Take your struggle in stride.

Yogananda wrote in his autobiography that the struggles of the battlefield pale in insignificance compared to the turmoil that occurs when man first contends with his inner enemies. I try to remember this passage when I fall out of posture, or when I'm struck by my own stupidity or appalled by my ugliness. Touching the struggles of our life with compassion is the real work. After all, it's just yoga. We're just a bunch of strangers sweating in a hot room.

If we can learn to take our struggles in stride during the postures, imagine what battles we might win off the mat. Where should we stand so that healing may occur? Right in front of the mirror, confronting our most significant enemy of all—our inner critic or naysayer.

 Even while you're struggling, will you create a force of kindness around yourself?

October 1

Take a small step, physically and emotionally.

Newton's third law states that for every action, there is an equal and opposite reaction. Yoga is no exception to this law, except the reaction isn't necessarily opposite. It might just come in another area of life instead.

For every posture in which we take a small physical step to strengthen our bodies more fully, we also take a small step in the direction of experiencing our emotions more fully. It's like the head and the heart speak to each other through the postures. *Hey guys, we just made a nice little chunk of progress up here in brain world, so please follow suit.*

And the heart does, every time. Yoga shows us that the physiological is the back door to the psychological. You risk going deeper in tree pose, and perhaps you take more chances voicing opinions at work. You open up your thoracic cavity in camel pose, and perhaps you become more vulnerable with your significant other. It's a beautiful dance that happens inside of you.

 Are you using yoga as the music to get your parts grooving together?

October 2

Tap into your inspiration reserves.

I once spent two weeks sitting on jury duty. The courtroom was cold, ugly, and harsh, and the deliberation room was stuffy, cramped, and boring. It's not exactly an inspiring environment to stimulate the creative juices, but I didn't let that stop me from doing my work. After all, meaning is made, not found. It's our responsibility to take control of our lives and make the most out of our environment, instead of allowing circumstances to dictate our happiness.

Every day I brought a briefcase full of work to do, books to read, projects to start, upbeat music to listen to, and other tools to maximize an otherwise dreary experience. During our many recesses, I set up my portable creative environment and found a way to thrive despite my surroundings. During those two weeks, my days were filled with joy and meaning and energy and productivity; I even learned a thing or two about the judicial system. Thriving in a difficult environment is always possible, but only if you are intentional. If I hadn't tapped into my reserves to create inspiration where none existed, I would have had a grumpy time of it.

It's like my yoga instructor always says during class: This is just practice. The real work is taking this yoga out into the world. It's one thing to relax in a studio, it's another thing to relax in the middle of rush-hour traffic. Whether you're trying to meditate, or whether you're just trying to create, don't expect the environment to do the work for you. Instead of only seeing the obstacles, give yourself the tools you need to flourish.

 How can you make the most of a challenging situation?

October 3

Distinguish between discomfort and distress.

Yoga helps you discern the difference between discomfort and distress. *Discomfort*, although it may feel unpleasant, is tolerable. Like when your knees are buckling and your muscles are pulsing, but you keep breathing and stay in the posture and trust the gifts that might accompany those uneasy feelings. That's normal, navigable, and not worth panicking about.

Distress, on the other hand, is overwhelming and impairs your ability to function. It might even require immediate assistance. Like when you're not properly hydrated for class and the heat is blasting and you push so hard that you start noticing little blips and stars out of the corner of your eye.

Distress does happen, but after thousands of classes and ten years of practice, I can only remember a handful of legitimately distressing moments. Usually those alarms are just fear masquerading as the voice of wisdom. So don't hit the panic button too soon. Take a moment to breathe and assess. Managing discomfort is one of the key abilities for persevering and making strides against adversity.

 How did you learn the difference between discomfort and distress?

October 4

Rescue yourself for a change.

Some people are addicted to being rescuers. Their drug of choice is the euphoric experience of pulling someone into a lifeboat. The irony, of course, is that the people they "save" never make it to shore. They always end up back in the water. Because deep down, they don't really want to be saved. That would mean they'd actually have to change, take responsibility, and surrender their victim position.

One of my yoga instructors also works as a sponsor for alcoholics in the twelve-step program. She often gets phone calls, sometimes very late at night, from people in recovery who have a difficult time changing. Often, she won't say a word in response to their pleas. Her job isn't to rescue people; her job is to listen to them. In fact, she has a great mantra that I try to practice myself: Sometimes you can't get people to listen to you until you stop talking.

If there are people in your life for whom you're tired of being an unpaid, part-time therapist, set the boundary of silence. Try not rescuing them and see what happens. Maybe they'll change on their own clock. Remember, you can't take people where they don't want to go.

 Who are you trying to rescue that doesn't want to be saved?

October 5

React wisely.

Buddha taught about a phenomenon called the second arrow. When we encounter something that leads to pain, we launch into a chorus of mental processes that lead to more suffering. It's the hardest trap not to fall into. Whatever negative emotional experiences we have swiftly infect everything around them. The second arrow manifests all the time in different ways.

When we're down, everything we do seems to come out wrong. When we're struggling, even stuff we love is hard to care about. When we're heartbroken, everything feels like a rejection. When we're overwhelmed, everything feels like a number one priority. When we're lonely, we withdraw from others. All of that is the second arrow. It's the compounding of an initial pain with suffering of our own making.

We even shoot that arrow at ourselves during class. Perhaps we hold a posture for thirty seconds longer than normal one day. Discomfort, frustration, and even pain increase. That's the first arrow. But how we react to that sensation, the second arrow, is what matters. That's our yoga for the day.

We can react by adding value-laden stories and judgments to a value-neutral sensation, or we can watch and wonder what those sensations are trying to tell us. Maybe it just means we're giving our muscles a chance to grow stronger, but we read it as a sign that our muscles are weak. The mystics were right when they said that pain is inevitable, suffering is optional. We just have to know the difference.

 What is your favorite way to shoot the second arrow at yourself?

October 6

Go to bed with a clean slate.

Millions of people battle insomnia night after night. Sometimes it's from a medical problem like sleep apnea, but often it's a combination of unhealthy bedtime rituals that interfere with quality rest. I do yoga with a psychologist who struggles with sleep on a semi-regular basis. Although he'd prefer to blame the tiredness on some mysterious and uncontrollable condition he's been stricken with, he knows that's just a way of abdicating responsibility. More often than not, his inability to sleep is tied to an obvious and temporary cause like emotional distress. As he says, insomnia is revenge for all the stuff you haven't given enough thought.

Now instead of counting cracks in the ceiling, he grabs his journal and follows his feelings to a deep slumber. Dealing with our situation by facing it? That's the best sleep aid on the market.

 What are you running from during the day that's keeping you up at night?

October 7

Steer clear of the brain through breath.

Monkey mind is an obstacle for even the most devoted yogi. Psychotherapist Eric Maisel calls this state *racing brain syndrome*. He explains that when we're dealing with endless thoughts and have no brake pedal, our behavior inclines itself toward insomnia, mania, obsession, compulsion, and addiction. Not the picture of health!

Our minds are always trying to distract us, jumping from thought to thought as if ideas were branches on a tree. The poet Yeats prayed, *God guard me from the thoughts men think*. But with so many questions and voices and ideas inside our heads spinning like plates on sticks, perhaps the thoughts of other men aren't our problem.

Despite the powers of the racing brain, I have slowly become skilled at quieting the thoughts inside my head during yoga class. It took many years to master this.

Instead of banging around on the endless racetrack of compulsive thoughts, I firmly turn my attention to the breath. As an alternative to trying to control and judge the stream of thoughts that runs along my mind, I firmly turn my attention to the breath.

Are you noticing a pattern? Channel those anxious, yammering neurons elsewhere. Spend your energy on a new pursuit, and the thoughts will go away. As my yoga teacher loves to say, the brain is a bad neighborhood. Stay out of it. Don't let yourself be yanked around by your thoughts. Turn your attention to something else.

 Do you tend to underestimate the extent to which your own hostile thoughts impact your life?

October 8

Accept your own imperfections.

We love to go on a mission to fix ourselves. We honestly but erroneously believe that solving all of our problems will automatically mean that we'll have what we want. Of course, that's not how transformation works. If we have any intention of getting to the next level, what we need is more compassion. That takes the willingness to see what is real about ourselves, without having to color, fix, or soften it.

It's hard as hell. Acceptance, for most people, is a scary way to relate to our own imperfection. The willingness to turn off the problem-solving part of our brain and just be with who we are, that takes practice. Yoga has helped me in that regard tremendously. Because every day, my body is a little bit different. Every day, my joints and muscles and bones and limbs tell a new story.

During each class, all I can do is look at myself through the eyes of compassion and accept where I am at today. No expectations, no judgments. This is it. This is what I'm working with today.

 Have you learned to be at peace with imperfection?

October 9

Activate the central lever that galvanizes the whole machine.

Commitment is the most underrated yoga posture on the planet. Staying focused and being disciplined while breathing deeply and finding your center all come naturally to the students who truly commit. They operate on a different plane. In their world they can't avoid doing the work, because they're not distracting themselves with anything else *but* the work. Everything else is white noise.

If you want to simplify your practice, treat commitment as your byword. The one-time decision that makes a thousand future decisions so we don't exhaust ourselves. The lead domino that knocks down all the others. It's more liberating than you can possibly imagine.

With commitment, you make your furnace burn strongly before you begin. That way, whether doing yoga or pursuing goals outside the studio, your progress isn't dependent on mood, willingness, timing, energy, or environment. Commitment trumps all of that.

 How are you laying a foundation that builds commitment?

October 10

Reject the concept of not-enough.

Hot yoga isn't a twelve-step program, it's a twenty-six-step program—one for each pose. Not unlike mainstream recovery work, it's a very human, vulnerable, and useful vehicle for overcoming addiction and compulsion.

Personally, yoga has done wonders for my own issues. For example, one of the harsh realities of being a workaholic is not understanding the concept of "enough." There is no boundary. Meanwhile, the people you care about most are left with crumbs. Remains of the day that trickle down your collar. To overcome it, we need to learn how much is enough.

Whatever your main stumbling block is, yoga is a practice that schools you in the concept of enough. You get on the mat and do the postures and listen to your body, and it will tell you exactly when to sit out, when to step up, when to take a drink, and more. As we learn how much is enough in the yoga room, we also learn how much is enough in other areas of life. We grow able to pause for savasana, thank ourselves for our practice, and step away until the next time.

 Which of your addictions could benefit from a new posture?

October 11

Be the couple that sweats together.

One of the best pieces of advice our marriage counselor gave my wife and me was to discover things to do together. Find overlapping interests. Be recreational companions. To get the benefits, my wife and I practice yoga together as often as we can. Not just in the same room, but really together. We make faces in between postures, we playfully pinch and poke each other, and we even give each other foot massages at the end of class. Plus, we trade stories on the way home about what kinds of feelings and thoughts and ideas came up during class.

It's strengthened our relationship in numerous ways. Because every class is another opportunity to deposit more love units into our account. No matter how good the relationships in your life are, they can always use a little extra attention.

 How has yoga deepened your personal relationships?

October 12

Retune your motivations.

Motivation doesn't happen *to* us, it happens *in* us. If there's something we need to discipline ourselves to do, it's not a question of making the time to do it. The secret is creating a rich context of meaning around the activity so it becomes existentially painful *not* to do it. When you do this, the time that is needed magically appears in your schedule.

Dragging our butts out of bed and into the studio is no easy task. But it becomes a lot easier when we change our understanding of what the studio means to us. If we started viewing it as more than just a smelly room to stretch in, maybe we wouldn't hit the snooze button as often. That's how I trick myself into practicing every day. My studio is more than just a place to sweat, it's a center of belonging. A neighborhood community. It's where I connect with people who have similar value systems.

That's just externally. Internally, it's also the place where I work out my emotions, purge my stress, and return to center. It's training to handle the demands of life, my antidepressant that keeps my sanity intact. That's much more motivating than feeling obligated to hit some external arbitrary goal.

 What is your motivation?

October 13

The exit is part of the posture.

Every yoga pose contains four essential stages: setup, transition, asana (or posture), and exit. In our laziest and most impatient moments, we often practice only the first three. After all, exiting the posture requires mindfulness, alignment, focus, patience, and understanding. After sixty seconds of twisting our body into a sweaty yoga pretzel, we're so tired and cramped and hot that the last thing we want to do is come out gracefully. In those final ten seconds, we simply give up. Our posture collapses. Tired arms drop to the floor and weary legs flop out like rag dolls.

Screech. This pose sucks. Where's my coconut water? I've been practicing yoga for ten years, and I still botch the exit almost every time in some poses. It's just too much work. Consider this excerpt from the instructor's dialogue:

Maintain your grip, abs engaged, keep your chin down, eyes stay open, exhale slowly, stay in control, push your big toe down into the floor, round up slowly, inhale slowly, keep the arms straight by the ears, turn ninety degrees, face forward, legs back together, exhale slowly, let the sweat drip, stand perfectly still.

Who has time for all of that? you might think. But then I remember what my teacher once told me: The exit is part of the posture. It's not some optional extra bonus movement at the end of the pose. It *is* the pose. How we come out is just as important as how we go in. Learn to come out of posture gracefully. Follow through with mindfulness, focus, and patience. The coconut water will still be there when you're done.

 What exit are you speeding past?

October 14

Welcome extra effort with a smile.

Angela is one of our community's veteran teachers. She excels in a variety of artistic disciplines, from dancing to singing to modeling to strength training. When she's not teaching yoga, she also works as an aerial designer for a variety of Broadway productions. Naturally, her classes are among the toughest. She works us to the bone. But she always does it with a huge smile on her face, and students never resent her for challenging us.

In fact, the harder she pushes us, the more benevolent and comedic she becomes. Like when we're forced to do an extra set of triangle or bonus push-ups between sit-ups. In between grunts and exhales, she will yell out: Love you, mean it. You just can't help but crack up. It's the perfect balance between working hard and playing harder. We could all learn from her balance of tough love.

 How many teachers do you have who make you sweat and smile at the same time?

October 15

Use your energy wisely.

Ralph Waldo Emerson wrote that nothing great was ever achieved without enthusiasm. It's very true, but we have to be careful not to become victims of our own elation. It's easy to enthusiastically plunge into a new project, only to realize that our ambition, intensity, and ability aren't sustainable over the long haul. Everybody wants to come out of the gate with guns blazing.

New students at our studio are often told, don't go for broke in the first ten seconds of the posture. You will literally burn out. One minute is longer than you think. That's the smart approach for doing almost anything. Relaxing into it and pacing ourselves. Without that mentality, we make ourselves vulnerable to exhaustion, frustration, even injury. Especially if we're not honest with ourselves.

That's a problem I used to have with my creative projects as well. I would become hyper-enthusiastic about launching something, to the point that I would bite off more than I could chew. The momentum would last for a few weeks, but it wasn't sustainable. After a while, I would just stop caring and the project would become a burden. No wonder I had stomach cramps all the time. There's a time and place to get carried away by our own enthusiasm. But life is a long game. If we're haphazard with our energy in the beginning, our aspirations will soon outpace our abilities.

 How effective can you be in inspiring others if you're lying on your back in a hospital bed with a stress-related illness?

October 16

The indications of our progress.

I once practiced at a studio that had the following slogan painted on the front wall above the mirror:

Sore? Tired? Sweaty? Muscles aching? Craving water? Good. That means it's working.

What a perfect mantra. Because in many cases, the elements that we judge as being challenging or messy or scary are the very indications of our progress. It reminds me of those old shampoo commercials. If you feel a tingle, that means it's working. Sometimes, we're just so used to sleep-walking through our actions that waking up feels strange.

 How did you first know that yoga was working for you?

October 17

Practice the infinite expressions of namaste.

The beauty of the concept of namaste is that there are an infinite number of ways to express it. When we smile and welcome or high-five first-timers at the front desk, that's namaste. When we move our mats so the people behind us get a sliver of mirror in which to see themselves, that's namaste. When we blow our noses and keep the crusty tissue in our pocket and not on the floor next to somebody's head, that's namaste. When we accidentally poke the person to our left and offer them one of those no-harm-no-foul smiles, that's namaste.

When we accidentally knock over somebody's water bottle and offer to refill it for him, that's namaste. When we laugh at our teacher's incredibly corny but well-intentioned jokes, that's namaste. When we give a round of applause for the newcomer who made it through her first class without vomiting, that's namaste.

When we introduce ourselves to that newcomer in the locker room and invite him to come back tomorrow, that's namaste. When we look the teacher in the eye and thank her for challenging us to reach farther than our known limits, that's namaste.

Every moment of channeling this spirit adds respect and intention to our interactions with people. It makes others want to be around us, and us around them.

 How does the spirit in you honor the spirit in others?

October 18

Release yourself into repetition.

Certain types of yoga (hot yoga is one) offer the exact same postures, in the exact same sequence, with the teacher saying the exact same dialogue. Every time. No matter where you practice in the world. It's a feature that often drives new students batty. They complain that the classes are boring, mundane, and repetitive. Our studio even had a few negative online reviews from guests who wished the series of postures was more diverse: Is this it? Is this all there is?

Well, that's a big philosophical question. But the answer is simple: Yes. This is it. This is as good it gets. This is the best day of your life. Learn to love it. Big wins often come from boring places. Even if the yoga seems mundane, there's value in the sameness. It provides you with a solid rock, a foundation, in a world that's constantly in flux. It reminds you that meaning is made, not found, and it's your job to layer magic on top of the mundane.

Most importantly, the sameness gives you a chance to practice slogging through boredom, and finding what might be on the other side. Erin Stack, one of my first instructors ever, used to tell his classes we could get back to winning the gold medal for being the most interesting person in the world as soon as class is over. For the next ninety minutes, accept and embrace the "boringness." You might be surprised what it holds.

 Are you willing to see underneath the surface of the mundane?

October 19

See yourself through new eyes.

Monica Felix is the studio photographer where I practice. She finds her yoga photography to be a form of namaste, a genuflection to people's patience and strength in their yoga. Not only that, she gets inspired for her own practice when she sees their poses through her lens. She also says that the secret to taking good pictures of people who are sweaty, half-naked, and bending in vulnerable positions is simple: You just focus on their eyes, their strength and form, and their sweat.

Their sweat? That surprised me. But she told me that students wear sweat as a badge, and it comes out in photographs looking like armor. And who could be ashamed of that? Too often, we get hung up on judging ourselves for things that come naturally, whether it's sweat or something else. But for an artist, those can be the keys to our very beauty. We could all benefit from a similar adjustment of our vision.

 Can you consider your practice as a work of art today?

October 20

Cherish the sound of chaturanga.

When the students in the yoga room become perfectly still and silent and all synced up, a whole chorus of beautiful sounds comes to the fore. The ticking of the clock, the dripping of the sweat, the humming of the heater, the flowing of breath, the popping of joints: this is the magnificent soundscape of human ambition. There's nothing quite like it in the world.

You can't bottle or sell it. Even the most advanced audio technology in the world couldn't recreate this sonic environment. It's unrepeatable and unbeatable. The more you do it, the more you start to crave those little sensory idiosyncrasies when they're gone. That's how you know you've found a home in the practice, and what brings you back to it.

 What does your favorite place sound like?

October 21

Let your thoughts come and go.

Freedom doesn't mean controlling our thoughts, feelings, and reactions; it means being in control of what we *do* with those thoughts, feelings, and reactions once they arise. We let go of policing ourselves; regardless of what we deem acceptable, whatever comes up is what comes up. It's not our fault. It's not who we are. It's just what we're experiencing right now.

After a thousand or so classes, my yoga practice has taught me to observe my mind and train it not to attach too strongly to the thoughts and feelings and reactions that pop up. Those thoughts? They're not even real. Only the action we take upon them is. Everything else is just a story inside our heads. There are no bad thoughts and no bad feelings, only healthy and unhealthy ways of expressing them. Once you realize that, yoga has liberated you.

 Are you free enough to be in control of what you do with your thoughts?

October 22

Embrace improvisation.

There are tens of thousands of yoga studios all across the country. But sometimes, busy schedules prevent us from showing up to class. If we're committed to our practice, we have no choice but to practice wherever we are instead. Over the years I have done yoga in hotel rooms, gymnasiums, beaches, patches of grass, steam rooms, even on the deck of a cruise ship in the middle of the ocean. Although it's certainly not the same as doing poses inside of a hot, cozy, modern yoga studio, it's better than nothing.

The hard part is not having any mirrors, especially if you're habituated to practicing with the visual guidance of your own reflection. But when practicing in an unusual location, you quickly learn that the mirror of the mind works fine. It may require a bit more trust and imagination than simply staring at yourself in the glass, but as any yogi will tell you, muscle memory is a beautiful thing. You may find that untethering from your routine even leads to unexpected revelations.

 Are you allowing yourself to be spontaneous?

October 23

Start strong.

The most important part of any class is the moment you walk through the door. What matters isn't what you do there, what matters is the fact that you *are* there. That alone is a symbol of your commitment, your humility, your willingness to ask for help, and your desire to grow.

Yoga is not about good or bad, right or wrong, win or lose. It's about being there. Woody Allen said that eighty percent of life is showing up. But I'd say that it's everything.

 Where are you still afraid to show up?

October 24

Build a new story.

I recently had a heart-to-heart conversation with a colleague whose business volume isn't nearly where he wants it to be. You could hear the fear in his voice. He even admitted that without the business, he didn't know what he would do with himself.

We can all relate to that struggle. It's a scary and vulnerable place to be. I've been there a few times myself, but the longer I stay in the game, and the more laps around the track I make, the less pressure I feel. Although I believe in my own abilities, I'm realistic about the future. It could all be gone tomorrow, and if that's the case, so be it. I'm a smart and talented guy. I'll find something else. Everything will be fine.

Saint Benedict, the founder of Western monasticism, used a mantra that I've always appreciated in this context: Keep death daily before your eyes. His saying brings savasana, or corpse pose, to mind. It can be the single hardest posture to perform because we are accustomed to always being in action, but it helps keep our minds and bodies connected with non-being.

Once you remember that nothing is permanent anyway, it's a refreshing reminder of life's ultimate end. Practicing savasana helps you relinquish your attachments. Our fear of loss is usually disproportionate, and accepting that everything is temporal goes a long way in reducing our anxieties. Sometimes we need to accept that we may fail or lose in order to become our authentic selves and see the truth: that who we are and life's value is not dependent on success.

 What are you still afraid to let go of?

October 25

Set yourself up for happiness.

Hot yoga classes are long, intense, sweaty, and exhausting. Sometimes you don't think you're going to make it to final savasana. But then that special moment comes. The one nobody can take away from you. It's the part of class where you're happy you came to class.

It's different for each student. Sometimes it happens within the first few minutes of pranayama breathing. Sometimes it happens twenty minutes into practice, once your heart is pumping and your skin is sweating. Other times it happens during a well-deserved cold shower after class. And sometimes it happens on the subsequent commute to work, when you realize that the hardest thing you're going to do all day is already finished.

Point being, happiness often has its own timetable. If you trust the process and trust the practice, it will show up when your body is ready to receive it.

 What's your favorite moment during yoga class?

October 26

Elevate substance over style.

There are almost as many styles of yoga as there are people to practice them. Here's a brief list:

Aerial. Anusara. Ashtanga. Bhakti. Bikram. Cannabis. Equine. Forrest. Hatha. Harmonica. Iyengar. Jivamukti. Karaoke. Kripalu. Kriya. Kundalini. Laughing. Nude. Power. Prenatal. Restorative. Sivananda. Snowga. Stand-up Paddleboard. Stiletto. Stripper. Svaroopa. Tantrum. Viniyoga. Vinyasa. Volcano.

Okay, that last one was made up, but tell me doing yoga inside a volcano doesn't sound awesome. Regardless of what type of yoga we prefer, the fundamentals are what matter most. Breath, posture, movement, focused attention, awareness: these are the elements that make any yoga practice special.

Alexandria Crow, a certified yoga instructor and educator, advises on her blog that we can't let the most vital component of the practice be obscured by its own packaging. The real substance of yoga, she says, is never the shape of the pose externally, but rather, the manifestation of a one-pointedness of mind, whether you're doing it on a horse or hanging from the ceiling. It's a powerful reminder that yoga meets us wherever we are, whatever name we give it. One choice of yoga style over another may better suit your lifestyle or needs, but the different approaches are all a means to the same end.

 What type of yoga works best for you?

October 27

Listen to the messages of the body.

How do you know which projects to focus on and decide where to invest your time and energy? Simply listen to what wants to be manifested. When you start working on something, scan yourself in those first few minutes of action to see which muscles and bones and systems feel tight, energized, or relaxed. Notice your breathing. Listen to what your body is telling you, and you'll have no doubt whether or not to proceed with a particular course of action or project.

I know, for example, that my anxiety typically manifests in my abdomen. In fact, recently I started working on a new project that I *thought* I was excited about, until within two minutes I felt pangs in my stomach. I calmly switched gears and moved on to a different project, one that created relaxation in my body instead of tension. This useful practice is something my instructor calls a *physical diagnostic*. It checks in with your body to see where you're at in this very moment.

Half-moon pose, for example, is a classic diagnostic posture. It comes early on in the yoga series, allowing students and teachers to feel out anatomical inconsistencies and gauge where their practice is at, for today. Whether you're sinking your toes into the mat or sinking your teeth into a new project, always listen to yourself. There's a message waiting to be heard each time you do.

 What are your bones and muscles trying to tell you right now?

October 28

Let silence work for you.

George Carlin was famous for telling his comedian protégés to accept what comes from silence. Make the best you can of it. Silence is the sign of the professional. It's true on stage, and it's true in life. Yet few of us have been trained to appreciate empty space in conversation or in our own mind. It's too uncomfortable for us. We hate silence because our anxieties get very loud in our head. Instead, our natural inclination is to fill any blank space with speculation or conjecture. To drown out the silence with our own wishes, fears, and fantasies. No wonder yoga is so hard for so many people. They're afraid of what they might learn about themselves.

Whether that silence exists at work, in the air at your yoga studio, or during a conversation with a client, it's something that should be welcomed, appreciated, and leveraged. Don't be so quick to rush away from the silence. Relax into it without urgency. Allow it to hold you a little while longer. You might be surprised what it produces.

 Are you letting silence speak to you?

October 29

Embrace the space between the postures.

Yoga practice is full of derailments. One minute you're doing the standing splits feeling like a superhero, the next moment you're slowly tipping over like a falling tree. That transition, that hallowed middle ground between stillness and posture, is where the real yoga happens.

In the web article "What Is Liminality and Why Does Your Story Need It?" Joe Bunting calls this *liminal space,* the moment between an inciting incident and the story's resolution. It is often a period of discomfort, of waiting, but also of character transformation. You can dread and avoid these derailments as threats to your serenity, or you can gratefully accept them as opportunities for growth. The choice is yours.

 How do you treat yourself in the moments between movements?

October 30

Let the sweat deepen you.

We all have an impulse to mop the sweat off our brow when we're overheated. Turns out, it's not a good idea. As each gram of sweat evaporates, it dissipates the heat into the environment. If you wipe away the perspiration before it evaporates, you short-change yourself from the benefits of the evaporation.

This happens in hot yoga classes around the world on a daily basis. We wipe our sweat, only to see it return five seconds later. Then we wipe it some more and it returns again. We can't help ourselves. It's just so annoying and sticky and salty. Seems like the right thing to do is to get rid of it, so we keep playing out this version of whack-a-mole. In reality, the best thing to do is accept your sweat. Even love it. When it's one hundred degrees and forty percent humidity, that sweat isn't going away anytime soon. Rather than fighting it, we must trust the sweat to deepen us.

The same process happens in our relationships. When we have people in our lives who drive us crazy, we try to wipe them off, to throw them away because they're activating us. But the moment we do, another person comes along and does the exact same thing. They trigger the karma that we haven't worked out yet. They show us the broken parts of ourselves that we still need to heal. The places where we get to find out what we're not finished working on. Sometimes we need to let things do what they came to do for us, no matter how salty and gross they seem.

 How do you respond to annoying things that have been sent to teach you about acceptance?

October 31

Set your own pace.

Yoga is a workout, but it's also a practice. A continuous and conscious journey that harnesses the transformative power of repetitive activity. The good news is, there are no rules for how many times a week or month or year we need to return to it. Our practice is tailored to our individual desires. Each of us shows up and creates a specifically nurturing habitat for the needs of our unique organism.

At my studio, some students show up every day, without fail. Yoga is the organizing principle of their routine. It's the iron rod in the center of their schedule. On the other end of the spectrum, some people can only squeeze in one class a month when the kids go to Grandma's house for the weekend. Either way, it's not about how much we practice; it's about how much intention we bring *to* that practice.

The unofficial first posture, then, is being honest with ourselves about what actually works for us. From frequency to pace to intensity, it's our responsibility to build our own personal yoga experience. How we do that is up to us.

 If you could create your own practice, what would it look like?

November 1

Find a way to serve.

My wife and I have been part of the work-study team at our yoga studio for many years. As volunteers, we participate in a special set of postures off the mat, including studio stewardship, by maintaining our beautiful yoga space; community growth, through digital and in-person outreach; and member services, by helping fellow students feel like family.

It's the best decision we've made in years. Work-study has helped us build community, deepen our yoga practice, and lower our monthly yoga expenses. What's more, through weekly tasks of doing laundry, folding towels, wiping mats, and cleaning floors, we've learned to embrace highly mundane and repetitive work.

That's the deeply formative part of working at any kind of retail space. There's always something to do. The work never stops; with a new batch of students coming in to practice every few hours, you can't walk away from it. The work may be boring, but it has to be done. Within the mundane is the satisfaction of providing a needed service. It's an experience that changes the way you think about stewardship, community, and the definition of work. Actions don't need to be attention-grabbing to hold value.

 What lessons are you learning off the mat?

November 2

Treat yourself better.

There's a direct relationship between how much we grow and how quickly we accept ourselves. It's not an easy task. It takes strength and honesty and courage to see the truth about ourselves with loving eyes. That's why yoga is such a useful endeavor. Through the bending and contorting and flexing and twisting, we literally see ourselves in a new light.

Whatever conversation we're having about ourselves or about our bodies, it's important that we rephrase it to make room for some acceptance. By extending unconditional positive regard to all the parts of ourselves, we grow. After all, the only thing that will bring us to the next step of our journey is accepting ourselves as we already are.

 How are you making yourself into the kind of person who practices self-acceptance?

November 3

There's no room for shame when we laugh.

At every yoga studio, fear waits at the door in a lot of shady disguises. Each student sees something different. Some fear the heat, some fear the stretching, some fear the teacher, some fear the advanced students, some fear the mirror. There are as many yoga fears as there are students to have them.

Personally, I fear farting. That humiliation runs deep. During a recent class, my worst fears came true. I accidentally ripped one that was so loud, it could have ended a marriage. It was hall of fame material. Talk about wind removing pose.

Funnily enough, nobody died. Everything was fine. In fact, we all had a good giggle about it. It taught me an unexpected life lesson: There's no room for shame when we laugh.

 Are you willing to accept the risk that what you fear might come about?

November 4

Thank yourself for being on the mat.

In *The Empire Strikes Back*, Yoda memorably tells his Jedi apprentice, "Do, or do not. There is no try." The same thing applies in yoga. When you get on the mat, you're either in the posture or you're not. You're either doing the work or you're not. There's no in-between. Even if it's only the setup of the pose, that's still yoga.

No matter how strong, deep, balanced, graceful, or ridiculous you look in the practice, there's still one thing nobody can take away from you: the feeling of respect for yourself for making the effort. Even after the most pathetic class of the year, you can still walk back into the locker room with the knowledge that you showed up and did it. Not tried it, but *did* it. Well done, Jedi.

 What are the efforts that are important in your life?

November 5

Throw yourself into action.

Where the eyes go, the body follows. Simply by lowering your gaze from the wall to the floor, you automatically advance a posture. Your eyes have just signaled to your brain that you can maintain balance if you extend further.

In the self-improvement world, however, you're told that where the mind goes, the body follows. That you can hope your way into progress by imagining an outcome. The reality is, thinking about something doesn't make it exist, only purposeful action does. If you're struggling to get your business off the ground or launch a new service or start a new creative project, forget about your mindset. Lead with your actions. Throw yourself into a tension that necessitates some kind of action. Paint yourself into a corner that you have to execute your way out of.

I witnessed this phenomenon firsthand when I began performing music in public. Busking under a tunnel forced me to sing and move and strum and perform in ways that were profoundly more physical than playing guitar quietly in my bedroom. After a few months, my entire approach to performing music and connecting with audiences transformed. All because I led by taking the physical action of going out in public.

Life rewards execution, not ideation. Go ahead and lead with your eyes in yoga class. Then once you get off the mat, let your body call the shots. Once you've made yourself physically closer to your goals, the rest will follow.

 How can you bring yourself closer to your dreams with action?

November 6

Tight pants versus light attitudes.

Yoga isn't just about fitness. Substance addiction centers are using yoga to creatively treat patients with mental idiosyncrasies that traditional medicine can't fully measure or treat.

The nurse who spearheaded the efforts acted on research that found yoga to be effective in reducing relapse, withdrawal symptoms, and even cravings, adapting support group meetings to incorporate yoga postures and philosophies into the process. She said, "Introducing yoga to my patients wasn't about dimming the lights, donning mala beads, and having people lay on the floor of the group therapy room. It was more about acceptance, having a sense of humor with themselves."

It's a sobering reminder that doing yoga isn't about wearing tight pants, it's about wielding light attitudes. We can do deep work when we look past the lifestyle branding of our fitness regime to see its potential to be life changing.

 What has yoga unexpectedly helped you heal?

November 7

Change how you experience time.

Albert Einstein's theory of relativity transformed theoretical physics and astronomy. Although the science behind the theory can seem complex and overwhelming, Einstein explained it with a simple metaphor: Put your hand on a hot stove for a minute, and it seems like an hour; sit with your beloved for an hour, and it seems like a minute. It's actually an encouraging approach to living. Einstein's theory suggests that *we* are where time comes from, and we can make as much of it as we want.

If I hustle into a hundred-degree room overflowing with a sense of dread and negative expectation, wishing I were somewhere else the whole time, *that* class is going to feel like an eternity. Postures will take forever. The hands on the clock will move in reverse. My instructor's words will come in slow motion. And ninety minutes will feel like ninety days.

On the other hand, if I walk into the room calm and hydrated and happy and emptied of expectation, prepared to relax into the space around me, time will whisk by like the summer wind. Even if I do glance at the clock, I'll notice that time has leaped forward in great spurts. The class will be over before I even know it. Because time shrinks and expands according to our mood, our experience all depends on how we choose to occupy the space we find ourselves in.

 How does your relationship with time affect your daily life?

November 8

Make sure to look after yourself.

A woman at my studio works the graveyard shift for the local police department. When she rolls in for the early-morning class, it means she just completed a twelve-hour shift, keeping the streets safe in the biggest city in the country.

It's no wonder she does yoga every day. When you work with kidnappings, violence, sexual assault, and human trafficking each time you go to the office, the workload wears heavy on your mind, body, and soul. I can't imagine how hard it must be to avoid slipping into anger, bitterness, and paranoia when surrounded by what she encounters.

So she practices every day to help. Releasing the anxiety from her mind, sweating the trauma she would otherwise store in her body, and gifting herself the same kind of care she offers to the city. To protect and serve starts with herself.

 Are you taking responsibility for meeting your own needs?

November 9

Treat yourself as you wish to be treated.

Every time you perform a posture, you reckon with reality and align yourself with things that will never lie to you, like gravity and biology. Some days, you can barely lift your knee to your chest, feeling like an inflexible failure. But other days, you can twist your legs into a pretzel like an Olympic competitor and you feel like a champion.

Either way, you must always love yourself. Confront yourself without condemning what you see. No need to beat yourself up when you make a mistake. Life will do that for you—our job isn't to help it out. And tomorrow, you'll be back on the mat, doing the work again.

 How do you get beyond your judgmental attitudes?

November 10

True joy is a serious thing.

When I was on jury duty, I learned that one of the most common types of lawsuit damages is called the *loss of ability to enjoy life.* Unlike damages for pain and suffering, which compensate plaintiffs for the physical pain they feel, loss of enjoyment damages compensate for the things they can no longer do because of the pain they are feeling, like playing sports or participating in their favorite hobbies. Consider what it means that our country's legal system values pleasure so highly that losing it requires compensation.

Do we value our ability to enjoy life while we have it? Or only when it's gone? If the latter, we can seize this moment to renew our thirst for joy. I used to practice yoga with a guy who moaned in the shower. Loudly, forcefully, and repeatedly. To the point that the other guys in the locker room wondered if he was hurt. It turns out, he just really loved showering. Especially after sweating it out for ninety minutes in the hot room, standing under a stream of cold water and releasing a guttural moan was one of life's simple pleasures. He wasn't ashamed of manifesting that delight for everyone to hear.

Americans hold it in, he used to say. Africans let it out. He was a beautiful example of somebody who doesn't complicate the purity of his enjoyment. Now follow his lead. Enough postponing your happiness.

 Do you make it a habit to enjoy life's pleasures?

November 11

Trust the floor to support your body weight.

Savasana is many a yoga student's favorite posture. There's nothing to bend or stretch or compress or hold. You allow your body to recover from any physical stress brought on from previous poses, giving it a chance to rejuvenate. Sweet, glorious relaxation.

Yet savasana is a surprisingly difficult pose to master. In the absence of a physical challenge, your brain and your body begin searching for little projects, like wiping sweat and shuffling your legs and adjusting your costume. Then, your mind starts churning with to-do lists. We struggle against the silence. In fact, there's even a name for it. Patanjali's sacred Hindu texts—the Yoga Sutras—named this phenomenon *chitta vritti*, meaning "mind chatter" or "whirling consciousness": the tendency of our brains to flutter from one thought to the next, and our bodies to fidget. Some call it "monkey mind." During savasana, our job is to release our muscles, but also to let those endless thoughts go. My yoga instructor often puts it this way: Surrender yourself and trust the floor to support your body weight.

In fact, sometimes he even encourages us to picture our skin melting into the floor. Surrendering our bodies to the floor below us isn't so dissimilar to surrendering our thoughts. Our actions don't gain extra strength by being ruminated over twenty times before we take them. If we trust that everything will work out—that not only the floor, but the future, will meet and support us—then we can start to let our thoughts go one way, while we stay rooted in place.

 What will be possible to you once you stop resisting stillness?

November 12

Trust your path.

Meditation instructors often implore their students to keep quiet about their practice and not to tell anyone they're meditating for the first few years. It's a boundary that honors the practice by keeping the energy and excitement inside until it's ready to be released into the world.

Without this form of containment, we allow the opinions of others to supersede what we think. We allow other people's doubts to weaken our faith before it has had the opportunity to mature. And that can hurt our journey in the long run. Because in the early stages of any new practice, you're damned either way. A lack of enthusiasm from other people can derail you, but too much enthusiasm from other people can prematurely give you a reward for something you haven't finished yet.

Whether it's meditation or exercise, diet or developing an unconventional belief system, the ultimate goal is to make personal choices divorced from the norms of the surrounding culture. While the foundation of your new lifestyle is still flimsy and unripe, don't be too eager to throw open the doors and welcome comments from all corners. When the time is right, you'll be ready to tell the world.

 What have you been incubating in your silence?

November 13

Access the frontiers of your mind.

B.K.S. Iyengar is considered the father of modern yoga. He has been credited with popularizing the practice, first in the East and then around the world. One of his popular quotations is a favorite of mine: Yoga is the master key that unlocks the frontiers of the mind.

Iyengar wanted his students to know that we can liberate tremendous untapped resources within ourselves. Through our yoga practice, we can follow his example and prove him right. In my ten years of practicing, yoga has been the key to locked places inside of me. Doing the postures lifts my spirits and opens me to deeper emotional, physical, and spiritual experiences.

Vulnerability, humility, sexuality, flexibility, compassion, acceptance, forgiveness, strength: whatever you want to access. Each of these resources had been with me always, awaiting my realization of them. That's one hell of a skeleton key.

 What is waiting to be found within you?

November 14

Look beyond the illusions that masquerade as reality.

The problem with playing the comparison game is that most people are posing. They make themselves and their successes seem bigger than they really are. Our image of their happiness is purely speculation. Edgar Allan Poe and Benjamin Franklin remarked that people should believe half of what they see and none of what they hear. Well—one of them said it, anyway. Different sources attribute the quote to each of them. Yet another reminder that nobody knows anything. We're all just guessing.

Consider the following phrase: Objects in the mirror are closer than they appear. It's the standard safety warning that's engraved on all passenger-side mirrors of cars. It's not only to protect drivers and keep car companies from getting sued, but also to remind people that their eyes betray them. That the vast majority of reality remains hidden from their view.

If individuals are suffering over comparisons, it's because they are similarly mistaken about the true nature of things. Perhaps they're accepting other people's bragging at face value, and feeling bad at not measuring up. Perhaps they're imagining others are successful in ways they aren't. Both problems are based on misperception. As the owner of our yoga studio loves to say, when you start to feel bad about yourself, find the lie. Uncover the unreasonable expectation. Identify the beliefs that are hiding reality from your eyes. And start redrawing the map of your reality instead of imprisoning yourself through comparison.

 What perceptions do you have about other people's apparent success that cause you stress?

November 15

Use what works, and leave the rest.

My therapist friend has a very inclusive, approachable way of working with her patients. When she offers them her toolbox for improving their mental state of being, she always reminds them to use what works, and leave the rest.

I love that. It's personal, it's solution-oriented, and it makes the healing process easier to digest. It's a great mantra not just in therapy, but also in yoga. When we used to work shifts at the front desk of our studio, educating and checking in new students, we would tell them the following: You can buy the whole package without *buying into* the whole package.

That sales pitch let first-timers know that they didn't have to join the cult, drink the Kool-Aid, or even practice every day. Just show up when you can and do your best. It's a powerful lesson for students, but also for anyone in a customer-facing business. Students, guests, first-timers, and newbies must feel liberated to engage, without having to subscribe. Otherwise they won't come back.

 What tools can you use to show up and do your best?

November 16

Use yoga to facilitate your superpower.

Once you commit yourself to a regular practice of anything, people start asking questions. One of the common ones is, have you ever considered becoming a teacher? Why not take the opportunity to inspire people to achieve the same sense of accomplishment that you experienced? It's a perfectly natural progression. Every great teacher starts as a beginning student.

But for me, even after ten years of practicing, being an instructor has no appeal. The thrill of a passion often dissipates once it becomes a daily task, and yoga is too important to me for that to happen. I deeply value the ability to practice yoga in an amateur and pure way. Being a professional simply isn't my style.

That's one of the reasons I focus instead on documenting my yoga experience. My superpower isn't adjusting people's standing bow poses, it's seeing the holistic connection between yoga and the rest of the world. Hence, this book. That's my version of teaching. Each of us has a task we're uniquely equipped for. You may feel dejected because you aren't interested in the options people present you with, sad that you don't align with their expectations of what comes next. But it could just be that there's another path meant for you.

 How are you making your regular practice into something that's useful for others?

November 17

Don't just wait for class to end.

In the kitchen, a watched pot never boils. In yoga, a watched clock never ticks. Ask anyone who practices regularly.

Whatever you are waiting for, it won't happen while you are concentrating on it. Because you're not being present. You're not staying in the room. You're just waiting for class to be over so you can go home.

Yoga is about being here now. If you keep staring at the clock on the wall between every posture, it will feel like the longest class of your life. But if you return to the breath and focus on what your body is trying to say to you, time will fly by like a wonderful dream.

 What's your biggest distraction during class?

November 18

Wake up and find your possibilities.

Philosopher Martin Buber once wrote that most men preferred to forget how many possibilities are open to them. That's why the great companion of change is curiosity. Realizing that we have options, and choosing to explore them. We must practice thinking to ourselves: I wonder how this transition will shape me. I wonder what hidden benefits might lie beneath this mountain of adversity. I wonder what the opportunity for growth and expansion will be.

Framed in that way, change is less overwhelming and more an invitation to adventure. Especially if you convert welcoming it into a daily ritual. One of the practices I learned from my instructors is to repeat a single, silent question to myself as I do the poses. Ideally, something that interrupts the worry stream with wonder and that converts curiosity into controlled inquiry. My personal favorite is: I wonder what I'm afraid to know about myself. This question powers down my racing brain; frames my psychic energies in more curious, imaginative ways; and catapults me into relaxation and focus within five minutes. Every time.

By the end of class, I feel refreshed and energized, ready to take on the day and listen to what possibility wants to be written. We can always walk through the world with wide-open wonder. No matter how much of a beating we have taken in the past, no matter how many rejections and failures we have endured, possibilities are always standing by, ready to be awakened.

 Do you look at the sky and wonder at your place in the stars, or do you just look down and worry about your place on Earth?

November 19

Just walk through the door.

In any given class, it doesn't matter how many postures we do. It doesn't matter how well we do them. And it doesn't matter how sexy we look while we do them.

It just matters that we're there. That we took the initiative, overcame the resistance, and showed up in the room.

 How will you conquer your favorite excuse for not doing yoga?

November 20

Step through misery to find joy.

Recently my wife and I took a particularly swampy, crowded, and intense evening class. It was brutal. Sometimes the hot room has its own agenda. Once we finished, my friends and I slouched into the locker room to grab a seat, catch our breath, guzzle some water, and regret everything we ate for lunch earlier that day. For the first few minutes afterward, not a word was spoken. But soon we all lifted our heads up, took one look at each other, and started laughing. As if to reassure each other, thank God it wasn't just me.

That's a beautiful moment in the practice. Especially if you're fortunate enough to have a strong, connected community. Yoga is an easy way to make each other feel less alone in our misery. Each person we practice yoga with (and encounter in the world) carries a little backpack with his or her own misery in it. Once we open it up and vulnerably bring it out into the open, we quickly realize that we're all carrying the same things.

 Can you see the silver lining?

November 21

Make breathing your first lifeline.

When you're practicing in a hundred-degree room with forty percent humidity for ninety minutes straight, the natural inclination is to ease your suffering with water. After all, it's cold, refreshing, hydrating, and satisfying. But as one of my teachers loves to remind his students, water is your second lifeline, breathing is your first.

Think about it. When a person experiences a health emergency, the first thing the paramedics provide is oxygen. Nobody inserts a water tube up your nose. People need air. It's the source of all things. And nothing against water. It's a close second on the scoreboard of human survival. But you can survive for three days without water. Oxygen? Only five minutes.

So if dizziness, leg cramps, and dark thoughts come crashing in during yoga class, the smartest response is to breathe, not drink. No matter how much money you spent on that shiny new vacuum-insulated double-stainless-steel water bottle that keeps contents icy cold for up to eighteen hours. Oxygen first, water second.

When our suffering feels intolerable elsewhere in life, we're given that same choice. We can reach for a crutch to soothe our pain, or we can regulate and refresh and rebuild ourselves with lifelines that are healthier.

 What's your preferred method of medicating?

November 22

We are the teachers we've been waiting for.

I once practiced yoga in a beautiful studio that had a series of laminated signs along the bottom of the wall. They read simply: *These mirrors are expensive, use them.*

Encouraging us to look into the eyes of our own best teacher. All yoga is still an individual journey of discovery. The most powerful source of wisdom is within.

The more we practice, the more we learn to trust our own feelings, and the more we allow them to become valid to us. So if the teacher instructs us to stretch further and pull harder and push deeper, but our bodies are telling us to stop and rest, we should listen to the latter. Even if the teacher is standing right next to us with his hands on our feet trying to offer a helpful correction to the posture, our body always has the final word. We don't owe anyone else anything. This yoga is ours.

This is a habit that takes years to form. In a yoga room (or anywhere else, for that matter), the forces of power dynamics, social pressure, and herd mentality can make it difficult to listen to ourselves over the teacher.

After all, these people have been trained and certified and committed to the practice for twenty years. They know what they're talking about, right? Absolutely. But the purpose of yoga isn't to follow directions, it's to water the root of inner wisdom. To absorb new insight by soaking it up from the bottoms of our own feet.

Nobody else is responsible for giving us the direction we need.

 Are you willing to stand up for what you need?

November 23

Respect rest.

Even Olympic athletes have rest days.

That's comforting to me, even though I will never compete in any sort of global yoga competition. Just knowing that achieving my yoga goals has as much to do with resting as it does with the amount of hours spent on the mat helps me grow.

In fact, it's one of the reasons I supplement my yoga workout with diverse fitness routines, such as swimming laps, cardio on the bike, and weights in the gym.

These activities work other important muscles, heal injuries, prevent me from getting bored with the same old postures, and most importantly, allow me to return to the mat refreshed. This diversity is especially essential as I grow older and my body doesn't give me the speed, strength, and support it used to.

Ultimately, it's a form of self-care, and we all ought to have our own version of it.

 What's your self-care rest routine?

November 24

Don't hide from others.

Warren Buffett's most quotable piece of investment advice is, *You don't know who's swimming naked until the tide goes out.* Meaning that in a recession, the weak will weed themselves out. The down economy will reveal whose product is a necessity and whose business practices are sound.

That same insight applies to our inner lives as well. Because in many cases, we don't know that we're feeling something until we *stop* feeling it. Until the emotional tide goes out. It's the law of contrast, like the drunk who admits to his sponsor, *I didn't know I was an alcoholic until I stopped drinking.*

The challenge is, how do we come to terms with our emotional reality when we're still in the thick of it? Through a connection with another person, that's how. One on one, being naked and seen and known just for who we are, not worried about anything except this connection we have right now—that's the doorway to emotional truth.

It's the reason practicing yoga alone is never quite as satisfying as it is with a class or a partner. Without that encounter with an intimate other, it's almost impossible to get out of the water and into the light.

When I think back to the low points of my life, the ones that lasted the longest were the ones in which I remained isolated in my pain. Only when I reached out my hand and stepped into the vulnerability of being seen in my struggle did the healing begin.

 Is there a person you can trust to show you the truth?

November 25

Be the welcoming committee.

Every time we have new students in class, I always make it a point to personally welcome them to hot yoga, usually by jokingly saying, *Congratulations.* Because at the end of ninety hot and sweaty minutes, they're wondering what the hell they got themselves into and how in God's name they're still alive after such torture.

But almost everyone has a good sense of humor about it. Most people are glad they gave yoga a chance. And for those of us who remember our maiden voyage, we have compassion for those just beginning theirs.

My favorite part about connecting with first-time students is saying good-bye. Especially when they're sprawled out on the floor, nursing a bottle of coconut water, shaking their head in disbelief, I always walk over to them with a wink and say, *See you tomorrow.*

A sweaty reminder that we don't need guards at the gates, we need a welcoming committee.

 How do you extend compassion to first-timers in your community?

November 26

Schedule time for joy.

Discontent is a fundamental part of being human.

Every day we are swamped by feelings that threaten to drain away our sense of power and ability to make meaning. And unless we physically schedule time for joy, it might never find a slot on our schedule. We'll become blind to the very things that make our lives feel worth living, too overextended and overly exhausted to make the necessary space for it.

Yoga, for example, is one of those experiences guaranteed to provide me with feelings of comfort and delight and aliveness and meaning and connection. Because I get so much out of it, it's very rare that I miss a class. But that means consciously carving the time out of my schedule, and valuing my happiness enough to meet my top obligations to myself over my responsibilities elsewhere.

Make that choice, and when life presents us with the choice between a cup of stress and a cup of joy, we'll have no trouble choosing the latter.

 Which meaning-making activities are you allowing to be put on the back burner?

November 27

Intensify the energetic flow.

One of my studio's yoga instructors was a minister in another life. She often brings insights from the faith world into the yoga world; going to her class is like going to church. During a recent weekend session, she made the following observation:

We touch the most high when we reach to our side.

It means that if we want to connect with something bigger than us, we must connect with the person beside us. Maybe physically, by offering a high five or a smile between postures. Or maybe emotionally, by quietly dedicating a certain pose to someone we love who's in pain.

But either way, if we are to reach for heaven, it's awfully hard to do so alone.

It reminds me of the popular scripture, *For where two or three are gathered in my name, the divine is among them.* It's a powerful concept, whether we're believers or not, implying that only through our shared humanity do we truly have a chance at real magic.

That's why our yoga studio feels like a congregation to me. Our collection of practitioners who flock together is a gathering of souls. Together, we create an energy greater than the sum of its parts.

 When was the last time you had a sense of belonging?

November 28

Watch yourself become stronger.

There are hundreds of moments in each class to build our strength. The practice gives us a venue for proving our ability to ourselves and building our confidence. Each time we overcome our excuses for not practicing, we become stronger. Every time we push our bodies to the edge without going over it, we become stronger. Every time we fall out of posture and laugh at ourselves before jumping right back in, we become stronger. If we breathe through a cramp until the tightness releases or stay in the room for the entire class and finish what we started, we become stronger. Every time we let go of something we don't need but merely want, we become stronger. Every time we inspire the person next to us to get back in and try the pose again, we become stronger. When we remain in control even when we experience strong emotions, we become stronger.

It's an empowering experience. With that new strength, we can do things we could never imagine doing before. Goals you thought of as pipe dreams may seem more attainable. Everything is suddenly within reach.

 How are you using yoga to show the world the strength that lies within you?

November 29

Release for greater resilience.

A key ingredient of resilience is acceptance. Once we understand that everything in this world goes away, there's no use crumbling the moment that it does. The smarter response is to say to ourselves, well, there that goes; what's next?

A few years ago I pulled a groin at a costume party. Apparently my sexy dance moves were just too hot for one body to handle. The worst part of the injury was that for the next few months, I couldn't perform several of the postures in my daily yoga practice. All I could do was sit there in silence while the rest of the students enjoyed the class.

But the good news is that the injury forced me to confront some eternal truths. It reminded me of just how fragile my own body is, and that sometimes, in the series of life, you have no choice but to let go of the attachment to performing every posture. In the end, that made me a more resilient person. It grew my ability to bounce back from future injuries and losses, failures and setbacks. Bikram said it best: You have nothing to lose, because you never had anything to begin with.

 Are you inviting every opportunity to build your resilience?

November 30

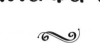

Get to know your feelings.

Most of us erect walls against our extreme feelings. We decide which parts of our emotional experience we're not going to have, and then, rather than face the feelings, we distract ourselves with immediate satisfactions. A TV binge session or adult libation, new purchase, or indulgence always beckons.

It helps ease our discomfort in the moment, but after a while, we start to pay a price for the things we're hiding from ourselves. That which we suppress finds a home in the body until our feelings transmogrify into illnesses, stomach pains, muscle cramps, skin problems, and other uncomfortable psychosomatic symptoms. A smarter tactic is to approach the extreme parts of ourselves in ways that allow us to be affectionate, not avoidant, towards them. To literally ask ourselves, What does this feeling want from me?

I often ask myself this question as a mantra during class, just to see what answers come up. What's cool about the process is that by fleshing out every last feeling I have about a certain issue, I reach a point where I have bored and exhausted myself with it. I express the same thing again and again and again until I have gone through it to the other side and there's nothing left to say. Once we've done that, we can move on. Sure beats becoming an accomplished fugitive from ourselves.

 What are you afraid to know about yourself?

December 1

Learn to respect yourself.

When giving thanks for the many benefits yoga has brought into my life, I count as a major one my new respect for myself and my body. Prior to starting my practice, I was much more likely to ignore or even deny my body's responses and pleas. That's what happens when you're a workaholic or a perfectionist. Your addiction to adrenaline and approval alienates you from your own needs. After a certain period of time, the inability to pace oneself leads to breakdown, burnout, and, in many cases, illness and injury.

All of that energy focused on achievement makes it hard to connect to activities that require taking a time-out from our goals. But the first day I tried doing yoga, there was a total body *yes*. It immediately helped me use my breath as the bridge between my body and mind, and it gradually trained me to trust my body to tell me when things were not right.

If you also have struggled to respect yourself enough to listen to your real feelings and to attend to what your body is telling you it needs, this practice may just be transforming your life as well. From only respecting external demands, we learn to value internal ones as well.

 Are you treating yourself the way you need to be treated?

December 2

Choose to build and nurture your community.

When we first moved to our neighborhood, my wife and I enrolled in the volunteer work-study program at our yoga studio. Not only to earn discounted yoga and free towels and unlimited water refills, but also to belong on a deeper level. It increased the social ties in our world and built a wider and deeper sense of emotional ownership in the yoga studio that we love so much.

That's how social capital works. To belong is to act as an investor, owner, and creator of a particular place. It's the opposite of thinking that, wherever you are, you would be better off somewhere else. Every time we return to the studio where we belong, whether we're taking classes, washing mats, drying towels, sweeping floors, or chatting with new students, we are in community. Every time we gather becomes a model of the future we want to create.

It makes sense, because the term *yoga* derives from the word *union*. That's the whole goal of belonging, the longing to be in union with others. This community, this place that we return to every day, is the container within which our longing to be is fulfilled.

 How can you assure that the experience of belonging isn't left to chance?

December 3

What's the correct posture for texting?

Occasionally during yoga class, someone's cell phone will ring. We always have a chuckle about it, because it's not so much irritating as it is absurd. The ringtone is like a bell of awareness for us to laugh at ourselves. *Wow, really?*

We are officially addicted. Remove our technology, and it's as if we've been cut off from our life source. The irony is, the promise of technology was that we would have more free time. Turns out it's the exact opposite. Peacefulness has been sacrificed on the altar of technological advancement. Even during something as relaxing as yoga class, we are living our lives kidnapped from the present moment.

Technology doesn't just do things for us, it does things *to* us. It's not the devices that are never off, *we're* never off. If somebody's device beeps during downward dog, don't scowl at the person. Ask yourself how *your* addiction to technology might make you act from your less evolved self.

 What distracts you most during your practice?

December 4

Make your transformation palpable.

Arthur Schopenhauer, the legendary philosopher, once said that all truth passes through three stages. First, it is ridiculed. Second, it is violently opposed. Third, it is accepted as being self-evident.

Yoga followed a similar path for me. Initially, my friends and family made jokes about my new pursuit. They laughed at my outfits, about the series of poses being nothing but sweaty stretches, and about me being one of three men in class. But once they started to notice the palpable transformation in my life, mentally, emotionally, physically, socially, the ridicule was soon replaced by curiosity. They stopped making jokes and started respecting me for trying to do something for myself. Some of them even asked if they could tag along with me for a class.

It reminds me of a brilliant saying from inspirational speaker Rob Bell, who said that you don't need to sell the world on the quality of your springs, just give others the chance to jump on the trampoline with you. It's a pretty hard offer to refuse once you see how much fun someone is having.

 Is your life a living testimony to what you believe?

December 5

Don't take yourself so seriously; it's only yoga.

The teachers at our studio work overtime to make the students laugh. They tell corny jokes, sing old songs with modified lyrics, do terrible celebrity impressions, even make goofy faces at us during class. It's like a game to see how many students they can get to crack smiles in the middle of postures. Not only does this make class fun and memorable, it reminds us not to take ourselves so seriously. To keep the practice light and embrace all there is to be grateful for with playful abandon.

In fact, anytime we laugh at ourselves, the muscles of the body lighten up, tension decreases, and we gain access to new flexibility and humility. We reach a safe place to try new things. Laughter can be an amazing medicine for all that ails us.

 Can you extract humor and joy from every moment?

December 6

When you lead with acceptance, there are no wrong moves.

The frustrating thing about growth is that it comes on its own terms and in its own time. It's realized at nature's pace and speed, not ours. We don't *try* to grow, per se. We simply accept ourselves as we are, and then we grow organically.

A few years ago, when my left wrist injury kept me from performing locust posture, my first instinct was to solve the physical problem immediately. I thought, *Let's get to it and heal this weakness ASAP. Then my yoga practice can get back to normal.* Turns out that was just me expecting miracles to happen according to my own personal timetable. It actually weakened my chances of finding a solution. Only when I accepted my body for what it was, not for what it might become, did my wrist start to feel better. Funny how that works. When growth is no longer our goal, we have more of it.

As you continue to evolve toward an ever more perfect whole, remember to be patient. You may not always accomplish things on your schedule, but you're growing and developing at the rate that's right for you. Remember, when expectations become demands, you're in for a world of disappointment. But when you lead with acceptance, there are no wrong turns.

 Aren't you just a little worn out from believing you have to control everything?

December 7

Focus on more than the party.

In hot yoga, the first twenty minutes is the warm-up. Only after we've done deep breathing, half-moon, awkward, and eagle poses are we finally permitted our first drink of water. That is one tasty beverage. This delicious moment is appropriately called *party time* at hot yoga studios.

As our teachers always joke, it's the shortest party known to man. It only lasts a few seconds before it's time to get back to work. That's the way it should be. As refreshing as the water feels to our profusely sweating bodies, it's not the most important part of class. It's just an accessory.

 When will you shed the next layer of worldly distractions?

December 8

Stand so that healing may occur.

Yoga may not heal us entirely, but it will help us establish a more constructive relationship to our problems. It gives us a safe space and the tools necessary to begin the healing process, lets us tap into and cooperate with our own healing, and invites others to support us along the way. Whatever brought you to yoga, the words of my first instructor are useful: Forget everything you read on the internet and just relax. That moment awakened in me a fearlessly compassionate attitude toward myself.

Pema Chödrön made a similar attitude the focus of her bestselling book, *When Things Fall Apart*:

> *I began to see that in some way, no matter what subject I had chosen, what country I was in, or what year it was, I had taught endlessly about the same things: the great need for* maitri *(loving-kindness toward oneself), and developing from that the awakening of a fearlessly compassionate attitude toward our own pain and that of others.*

Posture by posture, we can use this attitude to take slow and small and solid steps to build a forward momentum of healing. Humidity for our body, humility for our heart. And eventually, yoga will transform us. Remember, our pain indicates the lessons we need to learn. It puts us in touch with what we need. Let the lips of your wounds sing. Receive the gift of what's inside of your struggle. And believe you are strong enough to allow time to help you heal.

 Are you willing to use loving kindness to heal yourself?

December 9

Be a revolving door for your emotions.

Our emotions want to move through us. They don't want to stay, they don't want to be controlled, they don't want to be part of our bodies, they just want to move out. If you welcome them instead of resisting them, they will go away after being recognized. But if you suppress negative emotions, rather than accepting them, they can paradoxically backfire and increase feelings of distress.

It's like getting a cramp in the middle of class. You can jerk out of the posture, collapse to the ground, and rub the cramp until it goes away. But that reaction often creates more stress than it's worth and takes twice as long. Another option is to simply notice the cramp, send your breath to where it hurts, and ride it out. Doing so is surprisingly relaxing and satisfying and takes a fraction of the time. So it is with our emotions. Once we start practicing healthy *affect labeling*, or attaching words to feelings, we domesticate our emotions, instead of pretending they don't exist.

One strategy I find helpful is to keep a handy cheat sheet on my desk listing about a hundred different emotions, ranging from defensive to shocked to trapped. That way, any time I need to feel my feelings, I simply grab the list, find the label that best describes my current state, accept it, and then get back to work. It reminds me that emotions come and go like guests who come to visit. Some are welcome and we're delighted to see them; others, not so much. But in either case, it's temporary.

 How are you mindfully riding the ebbing and flowing tides of your rich emotional life?

December 10

Don't sit life out.

It's actually easier to do the posture than it is to sit it out. No matter how tired and sore and sweaty and frustrated I am, when I resort to squatting on the floor, slugging back water, and staring at myself in the mirror, it only makes me feel worse.

I end up just sitting there, feeling sorry for myself, with nothing to focus on except my own suffering, while time ticks by like a wind-up toy. That's when I say to myself, Look, I didn't come to class to not practice, so I may as well stand up and try again. Doing the work may be hard. But it's a hell of a lot better than the alternative.

 Are you giving up too soon?

December 11

Lay off the self-flagellation.

Rollo May's classic book *Man's Search for Himself* explains that condemning ourselves is the quickest way to drown our feelings of worthlessness and humiliation. As in: I fall short of the standard because I'm so noble and my expectations are high. In fact, I'm so important that God himself is actually concerned with punishing me!

I remember a period in my career when I would beat myself up for sleeping through my alarm. I'd think to myself, you're lazy and your life is going to pass you by. And then I'd spend the rest of the day—and night—secluded in a corner, working myself to the bone, trying to make up for lost time.

A smarter approach would have been to practice being kind to myself in small, concrete ways. Instead of leaping out of bed in a frenzied mess, I could have spent thirty seconds giving thanks for the extra hours of sleep that my body clearly needed. Instead of scarfing down a sandwich at my desk, I could have called a friend to enjoy a meal together. And instead of working straight until midnight, I could have taken a break midway through the day and practiced yoga with my favorite instructor.

Any of these strategies would have been healthier because they would have involved acting lovingly and generously to myself. But somehow, we feel more virtuous when we punish ourselves instead. Now? I'll take happiness over righteousness any day.

 Do you love yourself enough to stop beating yourself up?

December 12

Pick your battles carefully.

Most yoga studios have a "no cell phone" policy. Students are encouraged to finish their conversations before entering the room, leave their phones in their lockers, and honor the space by keeping the room technology free. In fact, I once practiced at a studio with a sign on the door saying that if a student's phone goes off in class, that person will be asked to make a twenty-dollar donation to the local food bank.

That's a bit extreme, but I understand where they're coming from. It's a respect thing. Students practice yoga to relax and reconnect with their breath and empty out their minds. The last thing they need is a vibrating device to disturb their meditation.

Still, we have to give people space to be themselves. Drawing boundaries is one thing, and being apoplectically infuriated when people violate them is another. Jean-Paul Sartre, the great existentialist philosopher, once said that hell isn't other people. But that's not true. Hell isn't other people, hell is trying to change them.

 Whom are you trying to change to be like you?

December 13

Don't rush.

During our first few yoga classes, we're likely to look at the clock repeatedly, wondering to ourselves, *When is this torture going to end?* But what we learn after practicing for a while is, we can't move through the postures faster than the hands of the clock will allow. That's part of the yoga. Maturing our sense of time. Learning how to surrender to the moment and forget about the clock. My teacher has this great saying: *Wonder when the posture is over by breathing.*

In other words, channel your anxiety into a more productive and present activity. Slip away from the domain of the clock by focusing on your inhales and exhales, and you'll float away to that lovely timeless world inside your body. No matter how far along we are in our practice, it's easy to slip into the monkey mind. Just remember, regardless of what the clock says, there's always plenty of time to listen to your inner voice.

 Was the clock ticking loudly, or was that just my heart expanding?

December 14

Yoga is just like ____.

James Geary's book *I Is an Other*, on how metaphor shapes the way we see the world, found that most people utter at least one metaphor for every twenty-five words. Makes sense. Metaphorical thinking is the way we make sense of the world. There are thousands of metaphors for understanding yoga, but here are a few of my favorites:

Yoga is like dating; you may need to try out a few different types before finding your ideal match.

Yoga is like life; there are some good days, there are some bad days, but in between many lessons are learned.

Yoga is like a spinning top; you go and go until you can't move any more and finally drop to the floor, motionless.

Yoga is like cleaning a dirty sponge; you massage and wash until the junk is released.

Yoga is like finding love; you have to be willing to try over and over again until you get it right.

Yoga is like daily existence; it's unpredictable and ever changing, but it's better than the alternative.

 What's your favorite metaphor for yoga?

December 15

Yoga is the sum of a million micro-corrections.

Small, quick, deliberate, and precise modifications may seem like nothing, but once employed, they make a huge difference in your practice. In final stretching, you touch your ankle bones together and flatten out the soles of your feet. In wind-removing pose, you lower your forehead to your sternum to stretch out your spine. In triangle pose, you lean your elbow against your knee to align with your shoulders. In standing bow, you lower the outer hip to get a better stretch in your leg. In camel pose, you place both hands on your hips to exit with integrity.

Each of these micro-corrections involves just millimeters of movement, but the moment we're teachable enough to deploy the instructor's adjustments, we instantly feel the difference in our bodies. Joints open up, muscles stretch out, postures lock into place, emotions float to the surface, sweat drips onto the floor, we're sore for the next two days, and then our postures are never the same again.

Who knew such a tiny correction could make such a massive difference? Personal growth is often a matter of inches, not miles. It's about our willingness to make a million micro-corrections, getting one percent better each day, trusting that the compound interest will eventually lead to a full expression of the posture.

 What was the best posture correction your instructor ever gave you?

December 16

Yoga isn't a competition.

When we finish a yoga class, our first instinct might be to ask ourselves, How'd we do? Did we have a good class? The problem with this kind of thinking is that it's trapped in the binary, goal-oriented construct of good or bad, right or wrong, win or lose.

But yoga isn't a competition. It's a practice. It's about showing up and seeing what you find that day. Instead, the question to ask ourselves might be, What did we notice? In our bodies and minds and souls, what came up for us? Those observations contain everything we need to learn.

William Shakespeare must have done yoga, considering his famous observation: "For there is nothing either good or bad, but thinking makes it so."

 How does black-and-white thinking distort your yoga practice?

December 17

Feelings won't be outsmarted.

Thomas Moore's book *Dark Nights of the Soul* teaches us that the soul's journey from misery to ecstasy has many important gifts for us. Even the most deeply disturbing episodes in our lives can become moments of transformation. Painful restructuring experiences that force us to alter our basic views and values for the better. The goal shouldn't be to give our all and move through our struggles in two weeks flat. That's only robbing us of the chance to learn lessons and endure through the important changes the pain can make for us.

Several years ago our yoga studio had a potluck. One student said something that affected me profoundly: "During periods of transition and threshold, the urge to hang on is really strong. The tendency is to try to negotiate a deal. To replace one process for another. But that's not transformation, that's just change."

If you truly want to lean into a radically different future, don't try to get there too quickly. And when you think you know your destination, you're often on the wrong path. It's like the hyper-competitive student who is injured and unable to practice. He's so anxious to get back onto the mat that he pressures himself to recover from the injury too quickly. As a result, he does a disservice to his body.

Moore reminds us that we don't choose the dark night for ourselves. It is given to us by life. Our job is to get close to it and sift it for gold. Knee-deep in a difficult period? Resist trying to resolve things too quickly.

 Where are you trying to force a radical change in your life?

December 18

Indulge your creative juices.

Within weeks of taking my first yoga class, dozens of new ideas and thoughts that I never would have come across elsewhere started pouring out me. It was much like how sweat literally pours out of my body during class.

Once yoga became a staple in my recreational life, the level of originality in my writing skyrocketed to new heights. It's as if someone unlocked a valve, I took a trip to another land, and my feet have never returned to the ground. You truly can't spell recreation without creation. Don't stress about how you need to put your nose to the grindstone to be productive; let your productivity flower by giving it space to breathe.

 Where do you get your best ideas?

December 19

Open up to true belonging.

College fraternities, underground clubs, and other niche organizations have a saying: From the outside looking in, you can't understand it; and from the inside looking out, you can't explain it.

This concept can be applied to a number of different communities, hot yoga being one of them. Because objectively, it's insane. The heat, the humidity, the length of time, the lack of clothing, the size of the mirrors; you'd have to be medically unbalanced to spend money on something like that. Yet, millions of people around the world do it every day. Many of them wouldn't even be able to explain its appeal to you. They just know they feel connected to something important via the practice. It's an important lesson that we don't always need to understand everything for it to have value.

 What do you love that you can't explain?

December 20

Put your energy only where it's needed.

The best part about watching competitive yogis is how they never make any tense, contorted facial expressions. No matter how strained they are on the inside, their faces just flap in the air like a dog's jowls hanging out of a car window. They have to relax everything they *can* relax. That way, all of the oxygen in their bodies can go to the places that are doing all the work.

It's a smart approach to yoga. A smart approach to life in general. Walk into the workspace of a pro, and you'll notice how they've arranged their work to coincide with their energy style. They spend as little energy as possible to get things done and strategically focus their available energy on the work that matters most. Walk into the workspace of an amateur, however, and you'll notice them investing all their valuable creative energy waging useless battles. They're drowning.

It's all about economy of effort. Focus on channeling your capacity for positive energy into the right channels, and while the rest of the world is nodding off in front of the television, you'll be left with undirected kilowatts to redirect into something creative and enriching.

 Are you focusing your energy on the right things?

December 21

Prepare to hibernate.

Sometimes we have little progress to show for a heck of a lot of effort. It's frustrating as hell. None of us likes getting used to the idea that we have to struggle to reach our goals. But that's the reality of any new practice. Whatever transformation we're trying to make, be it mental or physical or emotional or spiritual, will not come to us as a gift. We have to work for every inch of growth.

Yoga, after all, is a practice of minor adjustments. New students can't expect to perform the standing splits on their seventh class. Westerners have a hard time with this kind of thinking, as we've been primed for immediate gratification. If we don't get results from our new practice immediately, we assume something's gone wrong. We make the giant leap to global negativity. We've been doing yoga for almost four weeks or months and our body still looks and feels exactly same.

That's because sometimes, change requires a fallow period, a time when it works under the surface before becoming visible. Just like the seasons, our body may need a time of rest. If you're frustrated by a lack of instantaneous results, relax: it's part of the cycle.

 Are you trying to rush the future?

December 22

Finish with kindness to yourself.

We all are familiar with the final posture in yoga class: savasana, also known as corpse pose. It's widely known as the most important posture of any practice, and, in my opinion and that of many others, also the most challenging. That might seem strange, since students are just lying on their mats in this pose. Arms and legs are spread, eyes are closed, and entire bodies are relaxing onto the floor with an awareness of the chest and abdomen rising and falling with each breath. To the untrained eye, people are just taking a nap in a hot room with a bunch of sweaty strangers. What's the big deal?

Well, it's harder than it looks. Especially at the end of class, the reflex is to roll up your mat and towel, snag a bagel from the street vendor, and catch the nine o'clock train to make it into work on time.

The challenge of the final savasana isn't physical as much as psychological. We have to take time to give that gift of relaxation to ourselves. We have to believe that we are deserving of our own care and attention. And we have to accept that generosity and kindness without guilt, trusting that we are not the only ones who benefit when we love ourselves.

My yoga instructor once said we should think of the breath as an index of our generosity with ourself. After all, savasana is a safe haven from the whirling chaos and madness of the rest of the world. Perhaps the ancient yogis named it corpse pose for that very reason. To remind us to leave our attachments behind and just breathe.

 What generosity of spirit toward yourself arises if you slow down?

December 23

Keep following your path.

When I first started my practice, my intention was mainly focused on my respiratory health. Having just recovered from a collapsed lung, I needed a better relationship with my breath. Ten years in, my practice has evolved into more of an emotional experience. Now, doing yoga is also a daily routine of confronting and working through my emotions.

Maybe it's because the room is a hundred degrees. Maybe it's because I'm half-naked. Maybe it's because I'm staring at myself in the mirror for ninety minutes. Whatever the cause, after a few postures, any feelings that are present have nowhere to go but out.

That can be especially useful at periods when there's extra stress, whether because of the holiday season or because of one's own season of life. Come for the health benefits; stay for the more intangible ones. We all have times of the year that are harder for us; anniversaries that bring unwelcome reminders, or times when work requires your extra attention, or periods when shorter days leave you dragging. Use your practice to guide you through each challenging day, and the light at the end of the tunnel will appear.

 How can you use yoga to carry your commitment through?

December 24

You know you're a yogi when. . .

The comedian Jeff Foxworthy popularized the famous *"You might be a red-neck"* one-liners back in the early nineties. That formula can be applied to almost any type of person. Like people who do yoga, for example. You've been practicing for some time now. Maybe you have more compassion and internal flexibility from your time on the mat. Perhaps you might recognize yourself in the phrases below:

You know you're a yogi when . . .
You schedule your day around your class.
You keep at least one yoga mat in your car.
Your dream vacation is a yoga retreat.
You sweat while eating.
Your clothes smell like wet dog.
You no longer wear clothes.
You've used *namaste* as your email sign-off.
You become frustrated when some new person takes your spot in class.
You no longer freak out when a stranger sweats on you.
You find yourself breaking out into tree pose while waiting in line at the airport.
You're aware that the clicking sound in your shoulder stems from childhood
    resentment toward your stepmother.
You read books like this.
You write books like this.

 When did you first realize that you had become a yogi?

December 25

Give yourself a gift today.

What if yoga is harder than you thought? What if your practice isn't where you thought it would be at this stage in the journey? What if you're not making as much progress as the other students in your class? What if you can't touch your head to your knee yet? These are all fair questions. Yoga comes with an infinity of what-ifs.

But the answer is the same for each one: *It's okay.* Wherever you are in your practice, it's okay. There are no rules, there is no winning, there are no judges, and there is no finish line. There is only acceptance of the pace of your progress in becoming who you want to be.

Relax into your yoga reality. Believe that you are exactly where you're supposed to be, and try not to be so hard on yourself. The price of healing is accepting reality for what it is. If you can't touch your toes today, let it go. Your toes will still be there tomorrow. And the next day. And the next. It's only a matter of time.

 Are you giving yourself the gift of forgiveness?

December 26

Your body is an actor, not a reactor.

Some people have an external locus of control, and some people have an internal one. The former, convinced they are victims, believe they have little effect on the events that occur around them. But the latter have influence on much of what happens in their life because they're committed to the belief that they have an active role in deciding their own fate.

That's one of the surprising benefits of my yoga practice. Each asana strengthens my internal locus of control. My body becomes an actor, not a reactor. It's even been borne out in scientific studies. Participating in intense physical exercise contributes to real improvements in psychological well-being. Regardless of what kind of chaos is swirling around us, yoga reminds us that we control our reactions, shape our responses, and have the power to select the best path forward, no matter what may happen around us.

Though we all have suffered from various things in our lives, some more catastrophic, some more quotidian, it's vital to retain a feeling that we are still in control of our own story, no matter what forces are in play. Through yoga, we can seize control of our way of being in the moment. No one has the power to take that away.

 What accomplishments can build your internal locus of control?

December 27

Listen to your body.

Sometimes our bodies can tell us more about what's right and wrong than our minds can. Whatever arises in the body, we choose to greet it with a welcoming heart and accept it as a normal part of the life experience. We put our arms around it, thank it for stopping by, and ask what we're supposed to be learning from the situation.

It works in therapy as well as yoga. When you learn to love whatever arises, nobody can steal your peace. When you're willing to change your relationship to your discomfort, relaxation is never far away.

Next time your brain convinces you that something is missing, remember, your mind doesn't always know best. Listen to your body instead. It may have different, more honest information. Honor it.

 What are you listening to?

December 28

Your feelings have a beginning, middle, and end.

The moment our bodies experience discomfort, whether it's physical, mental, emotional, or spiritual, we immediately try to eradicate it. We rub it out or run away or take a pill or have a drink or eat four slices of pizza. If you're in the middle of cobra pose when you suddenly get a charley horse, your instinctive reaction is to jolt out of the posture and rub the cramp out. That's what we've been trained to do.

When I first started out in yoga, I would get searing cramps in the arches of my feet. I'd instantly roll over on my mat, trying to massage them out. But during one particular class, my instructor said something very useful: All of your feelings have a beginning, middle, and end. Her suggestion was to substitute massaging with breathing. Instead of interrupting your practice to rub out and relax the muscles in the affected region, try sitting with your feelings for five seconds. *Five seconds*. That's it.

I gave it a shot. When I felt a cramp coming, I just sat with it. Instead of freaking out, I simply accepted it, took a nice long inhale, and by the time I started exhaling, the cramp had completely dissipated. That's how feelings work, too. Whether they exist in the body, the mind, the heart, or the spirit, each has a beginning, middle, and end. When we're brave and vulnerable enough to sit with them, we discover they're not as scary as we thought. Yoga forces us to face our feelings. Even if it's only for five seconds at a time, it's a beautiful training ground for our lives off the mat.

 How has yoga taught you to approach discomfort?

December

December 29

Trust your follow-through.

The most demanding types of tasks are often ones that involve following through on an old project. Long after the mood has passed, long after you've run out of steam, and long after your inspiration reserves have been tapped out, you have to keep grinding. It sucks. You reach that dreaded point where you can't even conceptualize how the hell you're going to muster the momentum to catapult yourself out.

But just because your effort has been derailed doesn't mean it has to die on the vine. Entrepreneurship taught me this lesson, but it's applicable to yoga as well. We're not perpetual motion machines, we're human. That means we need to expect that there will be discouragements, delays, distractions, derailments, and disappointments.

And when that inevitably happens? We simply start again. We trust that we can re-engage with the original joy that got us here in the first place. Maybe we take a break or go for a walk before diving in again. Maybe we revisit our earlier enthusiasm. We don't need to feel guilty for fading as time goes by, but we do need to believe that we still have what it takes to pursue the goal we set.

 How are you bolstering your sense of being in the right place at the right time?

December 30

Open yourself fully to yoga's energy.

For all of the physical and mental advantages of yoga, it's also important to embrace the more intangible and mysterious elements of the practice. If you practice enough, there's bound to be some pretty far-out stuff that happens. It's worthwhile to share those moments, no matter how woo-woo it makes you sound.

I recall dozens of classes in which epiphanies and mystical experiences and other-worldly feelings came out of nowhere and rocked me to my core. In those moments, indescribable peace blossomed within me. The ground had fallen away and I was levitating. The flotsam and jetsam of my internal geography started shifting. Healing paved me like an avalanche of light. It felt like a wellspring of total-body bliss. I had transcended the boundaries of self.

These special moments can't be explained, nor should they be. Only notice and embrace them. Set aside any skepticism you might have. Transcendence can become part of your practice if you allow it to.

 Are you giving yourself permission to dip into the reservoir of cosmic yoga energy?

December 31

Erect a threshold between the outside world and your inner sanctuary.

At the end of each class, our final instruction is to seal our practice however we choose. Create a ritual that harmonizes your experience with nature, the instructor, and your fellow participants. It's a way to honor and protect and memorialize your work before you enter back into the busy hectic world off the mat. It also helps ease your fatigue and bring your circulation back to normal.

The fun part is that everyone has his or her own version of this. It's the most creative part of class. After thousands of classes for more than a decade in studios all around the world, I've seen it all. You can take a sip of water, fix up your space, bow to yourself in the mirror, rub prayer beads, take an extra-long savasana, do some stretches, bang out a few push-ups and crunches, pour water over your head, give your spouse a foot rub, recite a silent incantation, high-five your neighbor, make a mental gratitude list, exhale loud and long and hard, sing a series of ohm meditations, recite a prayer to yourself, honor the teacher with a *namaste*, or, my wife's personal favorite, fall asleep with your mouth wide-open for twenty minutes until students from the next class come in and kick you out.

Honor yourself. Thank your body. Respect the space you're in. It doesn't matter *how* you do it, only *that* you do it. Bow to your journey and reaffirm your steps along the path.

 How will you seal your practice?